Releasing Anxiety, Inviting Peace:

Small Changes that Make a Difference

Releasing Anxiety, Inviting Peace:
Small Changes that Make a Big Difference

By Elisabetta Reist

editor: Jeannine Norris

ISBN: 978-1501039157

Cover Design and Layout by Parry Design Studio, Inc.
www.parrydesign.com

Table of Contents

Introduction: Kiss Anxiety Goodbye!

"I keep the telephone of my mind open to peace,
harmony, health, love and abundance.
Then, whenever doubt, anxiety or fear try to call me,
they keep getting a busy signal
—and soon they'll forget my number."
—Edith Armstrong

D O you suffer from anxiety and panic attacks? Do you want to move forward and gain control of your own emotions? Are you willing to let anxiety and panic continue to make you a slave to their debilitating and tragic effects on your life? NO??? Well, good! This is your chance to take control and do something about these demons that have been trying to run your life. Now is your time to move out of prison!

I have done it. And you can do it, too. Are you willing to make a commitment to yourself and realize that you have the power to change yourself right in your own hands? If so, congratulations! You have just taken the first step to overcoming your anxiety and panic attacks!

As I share my story, I will share the steps I took to release the hold that panic and anxiety had on my life: how I learned what was causing my attacks and the tools I used to "kiss anxiety goodbye!"

Why Don't We Do Something About it?

So many people suffer from anxiety and panic attacks and don't take action. But action is important. If you remain right where you are now, nothing will ever change. And, again, I ask you: "Are you willing to stay in this spot and have anxiety and panic run your life?"

If living without anxiety and panic attacks is your goal, you need to understand yourself and your limiting beliefs.

I hope you are ready for change, although I realize it is not always easy to change. It is easier to stay in your comfort zone. You can then blame others or your circumstances for your panic and anxiety attacks.

When my first anxiety attack hit me, even the physician did not know what to say, and of course, was unable to help me. My parents were helpless as well and thought that I would laugh about these attacks once I turned 20. Why didn't they see that I suffered, that I was really in bad shape? What did it have to do with my age? I was 16.

So many people don't take action to control their condition because they don't really understand what's causing their attacks in the first place. I know I didn't. But we must learn more about ourselves in order to change our situation and to stay always anxiety-free. Wouldn't that feel wonderful?

If living without anxiety and panic attacks is your goal, you need to understand yourself and your limiting beliefs. Once you know what they are, and you are willing to release them, your life will become more rewarding. Imagine how wonderful your life could be without panic and anxiety. What would be possible if you were free from your boundaries?

I wanted to get rid of· my anxiety attacks and tried to talk about them with a friend of the family. He was a psychologist and was willing to listen to me. He seemed to understand why I was so frightened. His advice was that I should listen to my inner voice, to try to understand what it was telling me. I found out that my beliefs were keeping me from releasing my anxiety and panic. But now what? What should I do? Where were my boundaries and how could I eliminate them? Or was it better to transform them? Transform them into what? You see, many questions turned up. And I was still without a real answer.

However, I HAD learned something.

Where Does Anxiety Come From?

The first step in breaking free from the anxiety and distress that have been running your life is understanding what anxiety is, and where it comes from. You will then recognize the power of your thoughts. Yes, every thought you think has the power to either improve your life or to weaken it. The choice is yours. And there are many methods to release unwanted thoughts.

All of our emotions start with our thoughts. If you continue to *think* about the things you are anxious about— you will surely continue to FEEL anxious about them.

If your focus is always on what you do not want, you attract more of it. This is the *Law of Attraction* at work. It works in the positive and in the negative way: we experience more of what we focus on. We have to choose to focus on what we want versus what we DON'T want.

It is the same with stress. It's how we *think* about the events in our lives that causes stress. If you think in a negative way, your stress increases. If you can switch your way of thinking, your stress decreases and will disappear.

Fortunately, there is something inside ourselves that can help us. It is our emotional guidance system.

You will know if you are focusing on positive or negative things by the way you feel. Obviously, if you feel great, you are focusing on positive things. If your mood is down, you are focusing on negative things.

That brings us to a new step:

Change Your Thoughts to Change Your Life

The first thing to do is to quiet your mind. I reached this step by using Transcendental Meditation.

Transcendental Meditation, or TM, is a simple method. During a ceremony, you are given a holy sound. This is your mantra. You repeat it during your meditation sessions which last for 20 minutes in the morning and evening, usually before meals. Sometimes 20 minutes feel like hours, sometimes they fly by.

This method aims at quieting your thoughts. Whenever a thought shows up, you take note of it and then let it go. The thoughts that turn up are your stresses that try to interrupt your meditation. It is important to let them go. You will see that this method really helps you to quiet your thoughts and to quiet your mind. You will feel relaxed and even sleep better should you have a problem with insomnia.

This method became my daily companion for quite a long time. The results were quick and very comforting. The anxiety and panic attacks still hit me once in a while but they were less powerful. At a certain point they disappeared.

There are other methods you may use to calm your thoughts, including many meditations that were created by Indian gurus. There is also a simple method created by a French pharmacist whose name was Emile Coué. I have tried it myself and can confirm that it helps. He found that a simple sentence could calm your thoughts if repeated continuously. The sentence is: "Every day I am getting better and better and better."

When your anxiety mounts up, it is very important to change your thoughts in order to release the negative impact of stress. The above methods are all quite powerful. They can be used not only in the moment when your anxiety shows up, but also during the day, whenever you have a moment. They help to keep your thoughts calm.

Tools for Releasing Limiting Beliefs and Traumas

Becoming aware of your limiting beliefs is certainly the first step to setting yourself free and "kissing anxiety goodbye." Once you understand what is blocking you, you can release your limiting beliefs. There are a number of methods that you can use alone or in combination with other techniques.

Many of these tools are designed to help you release the energy blocks that are caused by stress. Everything and everyone in the universe is energy. There is no such thing as negative energy or positive energy. It depends on how we evaluate this energy. Energy cannot be created nor can it be destroyed, but it can be blocked and when it gets blocked, we can experience symptoms of disease or distress.

All of us experience events in our lives that cause us to feel stress. Stress can build up on a daily basis and have an immediate impact, or a long term effect. We have the power, however, to release this stress on a daily basis. It does not have to damage us. Some of the stresses can simply be transformed into positive energy that will help you on your way to becoming free.

One method that is growing in popularity around the world is EFT, which stands for "Emotional Freedom Technique." This method is simple to learn, can be used by everyone, and the results are sometimes immediate.

It helps to release limiting beliefs that we developed in childhood and that are still causing stress and anxiety in our lives. It is sometimes referred to as "psychological acupuncture" without the needles. You can learn more about EFT at *www.EFTuniverse.com*.

There is no such thing as negative energy or positive energy.
It depends on how we evaluate this energy.

Another method is called Quick Remap. It is based on acupuncture points, like EFT. However, other points are used that are even more powerful. For more information go to: *www.remap.net*

A third method is called Age Gate Therapy. This works on your spinal cord and on certain vertebrae. If you know when your anxiety started to show up, you may have somebody work with white light on the vertebrae connected to the age you had when your anxiety first manifested. This method can go back even to anxieties connected with your ancestors! In fact, the roots of anxieties and panic attacks are embedded in your subconscious mind. It is only the outcome that appears on the surface. While this therapy has yet to reach the mainstream of alternative therapies, it can be extremely effective and is worth investigating if other methodologies are ineffective in relieving your symptoms.

Anxiety and Low Self-Esteem

Your anxieties may be the result of traumas you suffered in your childhood. Abuses of all kinds could be behind them. And what resulted from these is most often a low self-esteem. Does this sound familiar? However, as you release the beliefs that no longer serve you, your self-esteem starts to grow and you learn to trust yourself. Events that used to cause you stress will be easier to manage.

In order to find out about my limiting beliefs and my low self-esteem, I started to search for my purpose in life. I read books, and attended conferences and seminars. I was insatiable. I would not give up as long as these panic and anxiety attacks continued.

As you release the beliefs that no longer serve you, your self-esteem starts to grow and you learn to trust yourself.

One day while I attended a seminar, which was not directly connected with my anxieties or my life purpose (or so I thought!) it suddenly occurred to me what my life purpose was. The seminar was about Feng-Shui, the energies that are around us. Energies that we can direct so that they help and support us instead of hinder us. We were doing meditations when I understood that I could give my time to other people in order to help them live a better life. It also occurred to me that if I had never suffered from anxiety and panic attacks myself, I would never have found my life's purpose. Isn't that wonderful?

I understood that everything in life has its meaning. Whatever happens in one's life, is there to help that person understand something. In most cases this "something" is important.

Don't Take Yourself Too Seriously

One of the best ways to reduce your stress and anxiety is to learn not to take yourself too seriously. Once I understood the power of laughter, I was able to laugh at myself and at the events of life. I was freed from self-condemnation and the anxiety that it brought.

We all have healing power within ourselves.

Yes, it is better to laugh, to not consider every little challenge that is happening as the end of the world. It is NOT the end. It might even be the beginning of your betterment. Be able to laugh about what is happening. It is easier to overcome the happenings if you do not think that they are a drama.

Read humorous books, watch comedies, laugh and laugh. Take a theater class as one of my clients did. Through movement and laughter and the exercises I gave him, he was able to heal a stomach ulcer and work out his stress on a daily basis.

Laughter is good for your mood and for your overall health. Did you know there was a doctor who healed himself by reading hilarious stories? He was seriously ill but, thanks to "laughter therapy" he was cured.

Learning to Heal Yourself Through Love and Forgiveness

You were born to be a healer for yourself. We all have healing power within ourselves. Did you know that? It is yours to be used. You can develop it so that it becomes stronger and stronger. You can heal yourself learn how to heal others, and even help others to heal themselves.

Healing is not only getting rid of physical pain, but also psychological pain, which sometimes is even worse than a tooth ache. Healing also includes finding the right relationships, getting a better job, or earning more money. All these things can be learned thanks to your healing power.

And the most important step in healing yourself is learning how to love and forgive yourself and others.

One day it hit me. I would only be able to "kiss anxiety goodbye" if I was able to accept myself. To love myself and to forgive myself. Many of us were taught that it was wrong to love ourselves. But we cannot accuse our parents for not having taught us to love ourselves. They didn't know better. They hadn't been taught it either. But there is no other way: we have to love ourselves and forgive ourselves. This is the most powerful step, though often the most difficult.

And once we forgive and love ourselves we can love and forgive others. I had to forgive whoever had not understood my pain and had thought I was imagining something or just wanted their attention. I knew that if I continued to think of the incapacity of others to understand me, it would continue to hurt me. I understood that nothing would any longer disturb me once I had forgiven the others.

You may feel that you do not want to forgive those who have been hurting you for such a long time. But it is of the utmost importance. We benefit the most when we are able to love and forgive others. Think of it: we do not have the power to change others. We can only change ourselves. We can choose to love and forgive others in order to help our own healing process. For more information on a wonderful healing process called Qigong, go to: *www.springforestqigong. com*

Love was meant to be the driving force of our lives. If you are suffering from anxiety, love finds no place. In fact, anxiety is the opposite of love. Why? Because anxiety is the absence of trust. So accept yourself. Love yourself. Forgive yourself for having allowed anxiety to enter into your life. Forgive those who hurt you. As you learn to accept, and love and forgive, you will learn to trust yourself. These actions will free you completely. You will no longer depend on the decisions of others, you will no longer need to be affirmed by others. You will be completely free. Your heart and mind will be in peace.

Enjoy the Journey

Your journey away from anxiety will be an exciting one. There are so many ways to overcome your anxieties, panic attacks or stress. Choose the ones that are best for you. You can be absolutely confident that you can heal yourself. But it also helps to have a guide. Someone who has been through it themselves, like me.

Life is not meant to be a struggle. We are meant to enjoy the journey.

I found my purpose in life: to help other people become free and confident. Free from anxiety, free to receive whatever they want from life. Confident that the Universe is supportive. This is the truth. It is your turn to learn it and to apply it. And you know what? If you want it, you can contact me directly and I will work with you on a private basis.

Life is not meant to be a struggle. We are meant to enjoy the journey. Life was given to us to be lived at its fullest. If you struggle with anxiety, you do not live it with joy. Are you ready to "kiss anxiety goodbye" and live with joy?

I hope you say: "Yes!

Anxiety: A Real Enemy

"Our anxiety does not empty tomorrow of its sorrow, but only empties today of its strength"—Charles Spurgeon

Congratulations for deciding to read this book!

As someone who went through periods of extreme anxiety, I understand that what you are going through is one of the most difficult things a person can experience.

I want to begin this book by validating the reality of what you feel right now.

Anxiety is an extremely unpleasant emotion, and it can come to you all of a sudden, or at a gradually growing intensity. More so, it seems invasive and all consuming. From a purely private and personal problem, you soon find that it can spill over your relationships, your work and even your health. Pretty soon, it just feels well beyond your capability to control.

What makes anxiety even more difficult to handle is that it is a diffused and subjective experience; half the time, you cannot describe what is happening to you nor can you explain where the unease is coming from. How can you then make the people around you understand something that they don't see? How can you make others understand that which you have difficulty understanding yourself?

A casual observer may be disposed to judge you for overreacting, for being too emotional or weak—or worse, just lazy and looking for attention. They will accuse you that you are just inventing a problem; that it is all in your head and you are making it up. And when they do, you begin to wonder if something is wrong with you and maybe you are crazy or defective in some way.

You are not crazy, and nothing is wrong with you.

I want to begin this book by validating the reality of what you feel right now. Anxiety manifests itself in many different forms and many levels of intensity, but it is a fact. It affects a considerable number of people everyday all over the world. And yes, it can paralyze you and keep you from the life you deserve.

Debilitating anxiety is a real enemy.

Defining Anxiety

It might be best for us to begin by defining what anxiety is.

Anxiety is a universal emotion. Almost everyone has felt some degree of anxiety at one point or another in their life. Those who have never felt anxiety ever are extremely rare exceptions—maybe they don't even exist!

While the signs and symptoms of anxiety differ from person to person, it is generally conceded that anxiety is a gamut of unpleasant emotions. The English word anxiety comes from the Latin `anxietas'` and/or `anxius'` whose roots mean `to press tight'`, `to strangle'` or `to be weighed down in grief."` It is a feeling of uneasiness and apprehension, usually about something that has yet to happen.

The effect of anxiety on a person can be felt in many areas. Your body can experience your anxiety through various pains and aches, stiffness of the muscles, nausea, vomiting, trembling, constricting of the chest, difficulty breathing and even tension headaches. Mentally, anxiety can be felt via confusion, difficulty concentrating, inability to remember, hypervigilance and obsessive thoughts. It may also come with emotions like anger, depression, irritation and fear of things like losing control or of dying.

Generally, anxiety is an unease regarding an unidentified threat; the feeling seems vague and indefinable. When the unease has a known target, the word fear is typically used instead of anxiety.

Is It Wrong to Feel Anxiety?

If almost everyone feels anxiety, does that mean that all people are problematic?

The straight answer is 'no'.

Anxiety is amoral, it is neither right nor wrong. As you do not choose to have anxiety—it just comes! —you cannot be accused of *full* (partial, maybe) responsibility for producing anxiety in your life. Anxiety does not come bidden, it is instinctual. There are things that we do, however, that maintain or intensify anxiety in our lives.

In fact, anxiety may be considered as a normal reaction to potential danger. Anxiety is a signal that there is the possibility of harm ahead, and that we have to protect ourselves either by fighting (facing the problem head on) or by fleeing (avoiding the problem).

As an instinct, it is likely something had been passed to us socially and/or genetically by our ancestors. You can imagine then that certain fears and anxieties have helped our forefathers survive. An appropriate fear of wild animals had probably helped them live without getting eaten alive. An appropriate fear of getting separated from the family— what scientists now call as separation anxiety for babies— kept young kids from going hungry when left to fend for themselves alone. These fears have kept the human race alive.

The same goes with us today. Imagine a situation where we are not afraid of dangerous things! We would just head on to high-risk situations with little regard for ourselves or the potential harm that may come to the ones around us.

A young girl not anxious about walking in a dangerous neighborhood in the middle of the night has a serious problem. So would an old man who does not get anxious about the health impact of too much of a fat intake—even when he is already feeling all the effects of a high blood pressure. If we do not have anxiety, we could die without warning!

The fact is, we need to be afraid of things that would not do us good or else we would not think twice about being plunged in consequences we do not appreciate. Viewed this way, not feeling anxiety when danger is already staring at you in the face is actually the abnormal reaction.

When then can we consider anxiety as problematic? There are three primary ways: when the anxiety is inappropriate, when the anxiety is too much, and when the anxiety is chronic and recurring.

Let us take a look at each one a little closer. The first sign that anxiety is problematic is when the anxiety is **inappropriate.** This means that a person feels uneasiness and apprehension even in situations where there is nothing to be afraid of, when there is no clear and pressing danger to self and others. It can also mean that while the fear is appropriate, its degree is grossly exaggerated.

When then can we consider anxiety as problematic? There are three primary ways: when the anxiety is inappropriate, when the anxiety is too much, and when the anxiety is chronic and recurring.

Consider as an example anxiety that results from meeting new people. Some individuals are so afraid of introducing themselves to strangers, that they avoid all social occasions and they go into profuse sweating at just the thought of striking a conversation! When you think rationally about it, what is there to be afraid of when it comes to meeting new people? The reaction seems to be extreme compared to the trigger event.

The best gage of whether or not an anxiety is inappropriate is to see your fears compared to the general population. If the majority of the population feels minimal to no anxiety at all with what triggers you, then chances are the anxiety you feel is inappropriate and potentially problematic.

Inappropriate anxiety is more likely when the object of the fear is psychological rather than physical danger. Fear of losing credibility, fear of making a fool of one's self, fear of losing self-worth are all real, appropriate fears that can easily become exaggerated.

The second sign that signals that your anxiety is problematic is when the amount of the anxiety is **too much.** 'Too much' means that the strength of the anxiety exceeds your ability to cope with it. The anxiety then already affects

5

your personal life, relationships and work life. It affects your productivity and your inner contentment.

When the anxiety is too much, there is usually obsession and paralysis. Obsession means that all you think about is the object of your anxiety and these thoughts just intrude on your day despite efforts not to think about them. Paralysis means that you have become frozen in your tasks and find yourself unable to perform as you should—in other words, the anxiety is debilitating. When this happens, the anxiety needs to be dealt with immediately.

The opposite of a debilitating anxiety is a facilitative anxiety; this is the kind of anxiety that helps rather than inhibits. For instance, some individuals function better when they are anxious. There are athletes, for example, who think that some amount of nervousness before a game gives them that extra adrenalin rush. Some people in business find that anxiety before a big deal helps them perform better, that it motivates them to take that extra mile. If you have been able to channel your anxiety in ways that make it more productive for you, then the anxiety is a functional rather than a dysfunctional thing.

Lastly, a sign that anxiety is already problematic is when it is **chronic and/or recurring.** If your anxiety has been around for a long time, chances are there is something unhelpful that you keep on doing maintaining this problem for you. Or perhaps there are new ways of coping that you need to learn. Usually, chronicity and pervasiveness are signals of seriousness.

Sometimes the object of the anxiety changes over the years; maybe when you were young you had a fear of public speaking but when you got older it became a fear of crowds in general. Usually this means that you are just transferring your fear to another object, but you have never really let go of the anxiety to begin with.

It would be good for you to do a little bit of self-assessment. Is your anxiety inappropriate? Is it too much? Is it chronic and recurring in nature?

What About Your Anxiety Makes it Extra Difficult to Handle?

Poorly managed anxiety limits the free expression of life and the ability of a person to grow.

The worst part of anxiety is not that it is unpleasant. The worst part of anxiety is that it can keep you stagnant and stuck.

All of us are meant to grow in life. The way our bodies naturally develop as we get older, so should our emotional, mental and spiritual life. This means that every day is a learning experience. When we interact with the world and the people around us, we get feedback from life on what it is that we ought to do to reach our utmost potentials.

And we are meant to experience life as FUN! This everyday learning process is not designed to be constrictive and forced. Rather, it is meant to be an enjoyable journey. A liberating experience. The way we can learn and grow in life is by simply using our natural inclination to express ourselves freely—without fear or inhibition! Life is not about suffering and hard work. Ancient wisdom tells us that we are born to enjoy life and not to worry.

Look at children as they develop. Toddlers learn about the world around them not from a book, or a particularly authoritative parent, rather from an innate curiosity to touch the world and figure out how things work. A young child would break a vase deliberately, just to see if it's breakable! He would vandalize the bedroom wall just to share what is in his head. He would speak out what is on his mind unmindful of judgment. As he navigates the world without fear, he learns what he has to offer the world and what the world has to offer him. He learns his limits also by exploration. And this is how his personality grows.

> ### *The more you think about anxiety, the more you get trapped into further anxiety.*

Whatever you are thinking results in a fact.

Debilitating anxiety stops us from exploring and reaching out. What it does is make us focus on what we are feeling, rather than what we can achieve if we take the risk. Anxiety is your enemy because it robs you of what could be your quality life.

While suffering the stages of anxiety, your only concern is to get out of the situation. Ironically, the more you think about getting out of anxiety, the more anxious you get!

The more you avoid anxiety-provoking situations, the more they come to you. And when you fail at managing your anxiety, the bad feeling just multiplies a hundredfold. This can be specially alarming as it is mostly the case that aside from the anxiety itself, people also engage in dysfunctional coping to deal with the anxiety such as drinking, taking drugs and alcohol or being hopelessly dependent on others as a recourse.

I understand if some of you reading this book have, not just anxiety, but a little bit of frustration as well. You must have all tried other methods of managing anxiety before and found that they do not work. This may be a problem you've had for a very long time. It is not unexpected that you may be a bit skeptical as well. That is alright.

I can tell you now point blank that there is a way out of the cycle of anxiety. But this solution would only come with a radical *change in your thinking*. You need to re-evaluate not just how you react to anxiety, but also how you approach life and how you approach anxiety as well.

While severe forms of anxiety are sometimes accompanied by other mental and physical illnesses, and thus require the help of a health professional and maybe drugs, the milder forms can easily be overcome with the help of the many techniques that have been known for ages, but mostly have not been known by Westerners.

These methods have now been simplified for use by Westerners or more specifically, by Americans. There are also methods developed by Europeans, Americans and other Westerners to help people who suffer from anxieties or other invalidating psychological diseases. Here we are going to explore several of these techniques.

Make it your own personal truth to overcome your anxiety. This seems to be difficult but you will see that it is a joyful journey.

And you will always be happy to have it undertaken.

Real Answers:
Nobody Needs to be Helpless
and Hopeless

"Happiness is not a brilliant climax to years of grim struggle and anxiety. It is a long succession of little decisions simply to be happy at the moment."
—*J. Donald Walters*

You always have a choice.

It is easy to fall into the trap of hopelessness and helplessness when one is battling anxiety. Indeed, anxiety is like a voice in your head that would keep on playing; telling you that you are not good enough, that you are not competent enough, that it is better for you to stay within small boundaries rather than explore the world outside. But at the end of the day, these internal messages are nothing but noise. They do not define your totality as a person— unless, of course, you let them!

It is easy to fall into the trap of insecurity, especially in our times. Modern living had thrust us in a world where, while we may have all the convenience of technology, we've lost our fundamental attachment to people and nature. It is ironic—in a world where we supposedly are more connected and more grounded, we are actually more alone and more ambivalent.

While the world urbanized, became big cities and towns, we lost the social network we used to have when we lived in small communities. Life is now hurried and driven, with barely enough time to sit down and get to know our neighbors and friends. Most of us even live far from our families, our haven and source of solace. Worse, with the number of issues family life is facing nowadays, divorces happening left and right, it is not unusual that there are moments when we feel there is the absence of a natural support in our lives.

We've moved far from nature. Have you ever seen a baby calf being born? Most of us haven't. Do you dare to spend one whole afternoon under a tree, just enjoying the breeze? Probably not. But our communion with nature is a huge part of our innate ability to be de-stressed. Right now, living in the modern city, the world seems cold and automated. By leaving our natural environment, we have anaesthetized ourselves from everyday wonders. We became purely thinking creatures focused on what to do next.

No wonder then that we have developed to become such an anxiety-prone generation! We have no source of security these days, no support systems and no known ways to de-stress. And while all these seem to be happening outside of us, at the end of the day it contributes significantly to our inner wells of security. The more isolated the world becomes, the more insecure we feel.

A New Paradigm

For us to be able to successfully navigate our way around anxiety, we need to expand our understanding and awareness of ourselves and the world around us.

Society, and probably our own upbringing, likely taught us that some things are more powerful than us in this life and that when faced with these more powerful things, our only choice is to surrender. Indeed, while we may not even be aware of it, we may be viewing our lives as nothing short of a power struggle—a competition to be the best, a battle to survive. Faced with a new challenge, we find ourselves asking: how can I conquer this? How can I be more powerful against this new villain?

In the context of anxiety, when something makes us feel terrible and afraid, our first reaction is to immediately rebel against it. If, say, going back to school makes us anxious, our impulse is to either squash the anxiety or find ways to attack the idea of going back to school. Our parents are too mean in making us go, society is too strict in its standards! But notice that the more you try to defend yourself, the more time, attention and focus you spend on the object of your anxiety. Soon, you find yourself trapped into fighting the bad feelings full time that you can barely think of anything else.

You need not view life as a powerful struggle. Here is why:

The entire universe is energy.

The world is not attacking you. The universe is not out to get you. The circumstances in your life are not in place to make you feel bad; it doesn't—and cannot—make decisions like that. The universe is a morally neutral entity. It moves but it does not make judgment.

Everything in the world is but energy; this includes the things that we see and even the things that we do not see. Our thoughts are energy, our body is energy, food is energy, our drinks are energy, and each piece of furniture is energy.

And get this: our anxieties are also nothing but energy.

Energy as such is neither good nor bad, neither positive nor negative. What it is, simply, is *what we think of it*. It is our *thoughts* that give energy a value.

This may be difficult to appreciate if this is the first time you've ever heard it, it is not a very popular idea. But take the time to reflect on it. Right now, think of your top three major objects of anxiety. What are the things that make you feel apprehensive and uncomfortable?

Having thought of them, make a list of the many ways you think about the object of your anxiety. What makes it terrifying? What is its effect on you? Make as many thoughts that you can about the object of your anxiety.

When you are done, go over your list and review them one by one. Chances are, you have come up with tons of negative things! For instance, if the object of your anxiety is dating again after a separation, maybe you've become anxious because you think you might get hurt again. Or maybe deep down you think you are not attractive and likeable. Possibly too, that you consider yourself as unprepared to go back into the singles market again.

Ask yourself now, *'Do I really have to think of these things this way?"* Are these things really negative or am I making them negative based on my thought? Is there a way I can view them, if not positively, neutrally

If we think of everything as energy, we know that we are in charge of changing its perception and therefore of how it will affect us. Do you choose to be affected in a positive or in a negative way? The logic would certainly tell us that to be affected in a positive way is more helpful and certainly closer to what Life is meant to be.

Energy means vibes.

Another important point to remember is that energy is never still and lifeless; it is always capable of influencing the things around it. Heat for example may just be confined in one section of a big room but left enough alone, it can heat up the entire house—even burn it to the ground.

Energy can fill every space of the world, every corner of your home and every cell of your body as well as every thought you may think. Related to the concept of anxiety as energy, this means that the more you continue to worry about your anxiety, the more you create more anxiety.

This makes sense even in neurological research as they say that our thoughts are organized in networks grouped together by feelings. Thus, the more we think about anxiety or something that causes us anxiety, the more we trigger anxiety-provoking situations. We lose immediate access to happy and content thoughts when we entertain the anxiety-related thoughts regularly in our minds.

Energy cannot make distinctions as to whether it is wanted or not, it just is. Consequently, the mere fact that we hold a thought in our minds can trigger the persistence of what we think about in our minds. Our subconscious does not distinguish between things that we "do not want" and things that we "do want". Thus, even if you know that you do not want anxiety, anxiety will persist for as long as you think about it.

Reflect about this nature of energy and anxiety because, if understood correctly, this alone can already produce a significant change in your life. It already directs you on what you can do to get rid of, or at least manage, your anxiety.

The solution to getting rid of anxiety is a commitment to mental discipline. We need to practice mental hygiene— that conscious and deliberate process of monitoring what we think about and filtering the 'dirt' from our thoughts. We need to eliminate that which causes our bad feelings, and get rid of the bad feelings themselves.

> *The state of your life is nothing more than the state of your mind.—Dr. Wayne W. Dyer*

Some of you may find what I am sharing a bit difficult to understand. Or maybe, some of you are even rebelling right now. You may be thinking: if it were easy to get rid of my debilitating thoughts, I would have done so a long time ago!

Fair enough. It is really difficult to clean your mind of obsessive thoughts—that's why they are obsessive to begin with! And I have no intention of oversimplifying your struggles. But I realized from experience that the difficulty people experience in removing thoughts of anxiety and objects of anxiety in their minds does not lie in the process per se. Rather, I found that thought control is only difficult the first few tries because we are not used to practicing control of what we entertain in our minds. With enough conscious effort, this can become second nature to us. The thing is, most people already give up after just a few failed attempts.

But with persistent and continuous efforts, the results are simply amazing.

How do we start this process of cleaning up our thoughts? It starts quite simply with an awareness of what exactly triggers your anxiety. Temporarily, you need to entertain thoughts of your anxiety causes just so you could to get to know what stuff you need to throw out. After all, you cannot change what you do not know.

So ask yourself, what is it that makes you feel full of fear? What causes your heart to pound so hard you fear that somebody could hear it? Are there many causes or many situations which you think are "dangerous" or is there just one? Is there a general theme to your anxiety? Make a detailed list.

If this first step of the process is too difficult or if you think that, in any case, nothing could ever help you to get rid of your anxiety, just let it happen and watch it as if it were happening to somebody else. Always bear in mind that everything is energy and that we are attributing it the value we think it has.

Once you know what you are afraid of, it is time to practice some techniques to develop your mental discipline. The following are three of what I consider to be most effective:

The Coué Mantra

We've probably all experienced what it is like to talk to ourselves. Even a little child, when he feels scared, assures himself: "Relax, calm down. Everything is okay." Somehow, these little self-talks can help "I know that whenever I tell myself not to be afraid of heights, all I am doing is making my fear more powerful than it really is. My fear is just energy and it needs to be re-channeled—not fed. I decided then to start telling myself everyday that I am more than capable of walking up a high ledge, and I will get better at it everyday. Now I am better able to look down from a high window without even batting an eyelash. " Megan, 33 console us and mobilize us into more constructive action.

A French pharmacist and humanist by the name of Emile Coué decided to exploit the power of us affirming ourselves. But he decided to take it a little further than simply telling one's self that it is okay. He developed a self-development technique called *conscious autosuggestion*. Also called "The Coué's Method" or "The Coué's Mantra", this method has been known to facilitate and cure for many concerns and illnesses.

One of the basic principles of Coué's technique is this: when you make a suggestion meant for your improvement, state it positively rather than negatively. Coué speaks of what he terms as a conflict between willpower and the ideas that we hold in our minds; basically the more you try not to think of something, or even not to do something, the more the opposite occurs. This is because the mere act of thinking about an idea plants it firmly in our heads.

This makes sense. Notice that if I tell you: "don't think about daisies!" you can't help but do the exact opposite—think about daisies! Our minds will form the image just because we've thought it. In a similar vein, the more we say to ourselves: "don't be anxious," the more we will feel anxious. In sum, Coué is basically saying:

Any idea exclusively occupying the mind turns to reality.

Thus, instead of thinking about the negative, or the problem situation, think about the positive—the solution or the cure. The best way to do it is in a relaxed way, not like you are willfully forcing information down your throat. The more a suggestion feels strange and foreign, the less likely will it take root. Coué suggests that the best way to internalize your suggestion is via a part of a regular ritual, e.g. repeating your key phrase every morning as you wake up, and ever night before you go to bed, and as many times you can in between.

Though you are free to make your own autosuggestion, Coué recommended that the best sentence to repeat every single day, many times within the day, is this:

"Everyday I am getting better and better and even better. Thank you."

You have the option of saying the above phrase out loud, or writing it several times over. While you do so, repeat the phrase as well in your head. Think of it over and over. By doing so, it can sink deep into your subconscious mind and help you to overcome an attack or the thought of being attacked by fear, anxiety or also by stress. It is a way of making yourself mentally healthy, like you are infusing your mind with the nutrients and vitamins it needs everyday until you get to the mental health that can fight off anxiety quite easily.

Relaxation Techniques

Our mind and our bodies are inexplicably linked, so much so that we can actually tell our body to feel better and it will obey us. This is particularly important as we talk about letting go of our debilitating anxiety. As anxiety can be expressed in bodily ways, consequently, we also need to teach our bodies to let go of its anxiety. A relaxed body is tantamount to a relaxed mind.

One great technique that can help our bodies to relax is called the Autogenic Training ("auto" means self). This method was invented by German psychiatrist Johannes H. Schultz. At present, it is used and found effective in a great variety of settings, including sports training, stress management and even spiritual formation.

In this technique, one is invited to conduct what Schultz calls as a body scan: mentally scanning our bodies for areas that are tense or not as relaxed as they should be. You may begin this by finding a position that you are most comfortable with, often it is sitting in a chair with your back resting against the backrest and both feet flat on the floor. It may also be done lying down.

You are invited to focus your attention on each part of you body one by one and "scan" it for tension, anxiety or even pain. You can go about it in any order that you want; you can start from your head, to your shoulders, arms, chest, stomach, legs and feet or vice-versa. Make a mental checklist of what parts of your body feels the most tension.

After your scan, you may begin inducing your body into relaxation. Mentally scan again your whole body, this time mentally tell the tense parts of your body to relax.

In Schultz' method, you are not telling your entire body to relax all at once, rather you will be doing it one body part at a time. Do not move on to the next body part until you feel a significant change in the body part you are currently focused on.

Autogenic Training works best with visualization---producing mental images of relaxation in your head e.g. a peaceful stream—and breathing exercises which we will discuss a little bit more later in this book.

An example of an Autogenic Training Relaxation Script is something like this:

"Breathe easily and slowly. Become aware of your shoulders. Move them slightly. If there is a tightness that you feel in your shoulders, let them relax. Let them rest comfortably against the chair. Now, feel that relaxation spread through your upper back... ."

The documented effects of these simple suggestions to your body are amazing; you would really feel replenished and ready to start a new day. If it is rest that you need, there are individuals who share that this technique helps them to fall asleep and wake up refreshed.

This is something that you can do everyday. It is estimated that regular training in this method for eight to ten weeks can already produce significant changes in your well-being.

For a complete list of exercises that you can do within the Autogenic Training program, Dr. Schultz's books on the subject are available in local bookstores and online. If you don't have the time to go through the whole program, you can just go through some of the exercises mentioned in the book or just what I shared with you. If you find a trainer with whom you can learn the method, it's even simpler and better, but you don't risk anything if you just do it by yourself.

Transcendental Meditation

Transcendental Meditation is a technique brought to us by Maharishi Mahesh Yogi, an Indian Teacher who came to the Western world and lived for a long time in the Netherlands where he passed away in January of 2008. His technique is very simple to implement but must be shown to you by a licensed teacher.

The meditation involves a mantra, a holy word and sound that you have to repeat in your mind. This sound brings you deeper and deeper into a meditative state.

TM is extremely easy to do because you get a holy sound and then you sit in meditation for 20 minutes twice a day, preferably in the morning before breakfast and in the evening before dinner. At the beginning, and this happens to everybody, the mind starts wandering around and doesn't stick to the sound given to you, but whenever you start thinking something else, you go back to the sound and do that for twenty minutes.

At the beginning, your anxiety may pop up even more often or get stronger. Maharishi explains that this happens because the root of the anxiety is being touched and eventually will be expelled by your mind. This technique is very powerful and helps you in many ways. It also improves your physical health, your awareness and then, what we are aiming at, the calmness and the disappearance of anxieties.

This technique has scientifically been proven many times and there exist various reports and books about its efficiency and help for people suffering from anxieties and also from physical diseases.

I would highly recommend you go and see a teacher of TM. The organization has got centers everywhere in the world, especially in large towns where they also have so called "Enlightenment Palaces". You have to pay to get the initiation, but then everything is free and you can go for multiple consultations where you can check that you are meditating in the way Maharishi told us to do. And you will always be welcome if you want to talk to some teacher.

How to Boost Your Self-Esteem: Various Methods That are infallible and Very Simple at the Same Time

"Low self-esteem is like driving through life with your hand break on."—Maxwell Maltz

Anxiety may be triggered by so many things that are happening in the outside world, but at the end of the day, everything comes back to the self.

If you know that you are a whole person rather than a broken individual, then you know that nothing other people can do or say to you can destroy your personhood. In like manner, no amount of difficult situations can ever take away your wholeness.

If you have that certainty that you are loved and that you are loveable, then you have that inner security that helps you trust in yourself and see yourself as competent and capable. More so, you also have that trust in the world that gives you the courage to reach out and ask others for help. You are not afraid that you might fall apart because you know that there are just so many people who can catch you if you end up feeling like you can't do it.

In this sense, anxiety is very much related to self-esteem. In fact, though they may not be aware of it, most people who suffer from anxiety suffer from low self-esteem.

Building self-esteem is not rocket science. If you want to strengthen your sense of self, there are simple but effective ways that you can do to boost your self-worth.

Defining Self-Esteem

The definition of self-esteem is very simply *self-perception*; it is in sum how you view and value who you are. It is a term used interchangeably with self-concept and self-worth. Family therapist Philip McGraw defines self-concept this way:

> *"Self-concept is the bundle of beliefs, facts, opinions and perceptions about yourself that you travel life with, every moment of every day."*

Some people perceive themselves negatively, e.g. they consider themselves as unworthy, undeserving and incapable—and thus the value they place on themselves is very low. Imagine a hypothetical auction block, where you are supposed to price yourself. People with low self-esteem are the people who would price themselves low—even free—because they think only `low' is what they deserve.

Others view themselves positively, e.g. they consider themselves as beautiful, loveable and capable. People who view themselves positively do not allow life to short-change them; they do not bend over backwards just to please other people nor do they allow public opinion to define who they are. They tend to be resilient, able to bounce back from adversity.

The labels that we put on ourselves are often learned. Usually, it is the people who raise us or who we interact with on a daily basis that form our self-concept. Individuals who grew up with parents who, from a very young age told them that `they are not good enough' or that `they should be ashamed of themselves' often end up internalizing these messages in their life. Parents too who are intolerant of mistakes and failure tend to develop low self-esteem in children.

Ironically, it is not just parental cruelty and coldness that creates children with low self-esteem. Those who grew up with overprotective and overindulgent parents also fail to develop a positive self-concept because the implicit message that being `spoilt' sends is that "I do not think that you can do anything without us." When you grow up in an environment when your needs are overly-anticipated, when you are not trusted to explore on your own and make mistakes, you do not get to practice your "life muscles."

Aside from immediate family, our self-esteem could be defined from significant experiences in our life. All of us have positive and negative peak experiences—those events in our life where we are most happy and most depressed. Intensely emotional experiences leave their marks on us. If we are not careful, a negative experience, such as a break up or a failure in school, can end up giving us a most negative opinion of ourselves.

The thing is, low self-esteem has no place in anyone's life. All people are born with value and worth, as well as an inherent dignity. We are all unique individuals with something new to offer the people around us. If you are a spiritual person, you know that you are loved by God by virtue of Him having created you. Our worth is innate—nobody can take it away from us.

And even though you have done things in this life that may be considered as shameful or a gross failure, your person is not defined by your shortcomings. All people can change, and what always matters are the choices you make today—not who you were in the past.

"Self-esteem is the fix that comes from the inside."

You have the right to a healthy self-esteem, and you should grab it.

Producing New Self-Perceptions

A simple way to raise your self-esteem is to make an inventory of your present self-perceptions. Often, we have no awareness of how we perceive ourselves. We may think that we have a high self-esteem but our actions contradict our belief. We may have to take a few quiet moments to sit down and really look at how we live and see if they reflect a healthy self-esteem.

List down as many answers as you can to the following questions:

1. Who am I?
2. What makes me tick?
3. What makes people like/love me?
4. How do I cope with adversity?

Dr. Robert Hemfield, author of the book "Love is a Choice", suggests that an indirect way of knowing your perception of yourself is to complete the following phrases with the first thing that comes to mind:

"All women are...

"All men are...

Usually, your list of what makes men and women what they are can reveal your hidden pockets of bitterness. When you know how positively or how negatively you look at yourself, you are already one step closer to changing your inventory for perceptions. You can assess whether these images are real or whether you still want them. When you make a decision to let go of the things that drive you down, the easier time you will have out of anxiety.

After making a list of your possible self-concepts, it is time you make a list of all the positive things that you do have. There are said to be three core elements of self-esteem, and the following are some guide questions that you can use to unearth them:

Confidence

What are the things that I am assured that I can do? Where does my self-assurance come from? Do I believe in my own potential; my capacity to overcome obstacles and achieve my goals?

Competence

What are the things that I am good at? What are my talents and skills? How have I used these things to make my life, work and relationships better?

Control

What are the things that I have the capability to change? How do I battle helplessness?

Changing Your Body-Image

Some of the easiest ways you can do to raise your self-esteem can be done in front of a mirror. Individuals with poor self-images usually could not bear looking at their reflection in the mirror or pay too much attention to parts of themselves that they do not like.

The different parts of our bodies reflect different things about us. For instance, they say that our foreheads are the repositories of our worries—the more wrinkles there are in your forehead, the more burdensome you feel your life is. Our stomachs are said to be the repository of our anxieties. Our laugh lines reflect how much humor we put in our lives.

Each part of our bodies are also said to have memories. Some memories are positive and some are negative. For example, our cheeks may be special to us because that is where our mothers used to kiss us goodnight. A scar in our leg may represent the memory of an accident. We need to acknowledge the negative—and use all the positives to distill our love for ourselves. If there are no positives, then that is the moment to promise ourselves that from then on we will replace the negative memories with positive ones.

Though we travel the world over to find the beautiful, we must carry it with us or we find it not.—Ralph Waldo Emerson

Take a moment and look at yourself in front of a mirror. Find out which part of yourself you dislike/hate the most and which parts you like/ love the most.

If you can, verbalize how much you appreciate each part of your body. For example, you can say "I appreciate my hands, they may be callused but they represent how much love I have devoted to my work." Affirm each part of your body because they are a huge part of who you are. Tell yourself that "you are beautiful."

This process is especially difficult for people who have a history of physical and sexual abuse. Alongside with professional psychotherapy to help process trauma-related issues, recovering your love for your body is a significant way to reclaim your self-esteem.

Gratitude and Forgiveness

Two simple ways that can lift your self-esteem and make you feel better are gratitude and forgiveness.

The ability to be thankful can go a long way in reminding us that there are so many things in life that we should appreciate. While negative things may come, these negative things are far outweighed by the positive things. The problem with anxiety is that it focuses us on the things that we do not like, when we are actually blessed in so many ways. The mere fact that we are alive is already a thing to be thankful for.

People who are capable of gratitude are people who have developed the right perspective when it comes to challenges that come their way. There is truth to the cliche "It could be worse!"

Try to make a list everyday of at least ten things that you are grateful for—the blessings that you have. Say thanks for the wonderful sunshine, say thanks for being alive, say also thanks for nasty things happening to you because they teach you something for your life. After a few days, you will start feeling better about life, about your thoughts because you get aware that negativity is no longer wanted.

More so, live everyday with a mind open for "opportunities to be thankful." People who actively search for blessings are likely to find them even in the oddest and the littlest of things, such as a quiet chat with the cab driver.

Let us rise up and be thankful, for if we didn't learn a lot today, at least we learned a little, at least we didn't get sick, and if we got sick, at least we didn't die; so let us all be thankful.—Buddha

More so, have a proactive approach to gratitude! Pass the joy around. Everyday, challenge yourself to create something you would be thankful for—and something *others* would be thankful for. A random act of kindness everyday just opens your mind up and leaves you no room for anxiety.

Secondly, practice proactive forgiveness. A person who holds on to so much resentment and even guilt are not powerful people—actually they are powerless people. They are actually saying that the negative feelings have much more control over themselves than they are, and that these feelings are too important to let go. The same logic applies to anxiety. If you cannot let go of your resentments and your guilt, how can you learn to let go of your anxiety?

Forgiveness is not a feeling; it is a decision. Some people think that they cannot forgive because the anger is still there. But it all starts with the mind. If you make a decision that you would already forgive someone—or forgive yourself!—then that is the point when you can begin to let go of your anger. You can decide to let go of your anger slowly everyday until there is no more. The less resentment that you keep inside, the more calm you'd feel.

Paul Scheele's Strategies

A program that I recommend you to consider is that of Human Development Consultant Paul Scheele. Scheele is affiliated with Learning Strategies Inc. in Wayzata, Minneapolis and is a specialist on the functioning of the brain. He has developed various audio courses, accompanied by a manual, on a great variety of self-help topics.

Three of Scheele's life-changing courses that I recommend are:

a. "Ideal Mindset"

This course helps you get clarity about what you want in life. It also provides easy to implement steps on how to get calm and determined. I think it is a very good help on various occasions in life, especially where low self-esteem and anxiety play an important role.

b. "Natural Brilliance"

This course helps you find your purpose in life. We all are meant to have a purpose in order to live our life fully and full of joy. Living our life with joy means getting rid of anxiety. The course offers many exercises that will help you find your purpose and eliminate bad feelings.

c. "Abundance for Life"

Abundance is not only material abundance but it tells us that our life can be rich in any sense, such as loving ourselves, good relationships, good health, material wealth. Here we also come to a central problem: most of us lack of love for ourselves. However, once we discover that loving ourselves helps us overcome anxiety, we understand that loving ourselves means loving life, means loving who has given us our life.

Other Natural Techniques

The following are other self-esteem enhancement techniques that you might consider for further research. These therapies are wonderful because they are completely natural, they use natural ingredients and the system will not be charged with toxins. In fact, your body will be freed from them.

Reiki

Reiki is a technique that originated in Japan and was developed by Mikao Usui. Reiki is an energy technique. You can give energy to yourself or ask somebody to give it to you. The energy not only calms your anxieties but helps you heal in any part of your body which needs healing.

Bach Flower Remedies

Among the many natural medicines that have the power to help your body and your mind are the Bach Flower Remedies. Available in most chemist's and alternative medicine shops, the so called rescue remedy can be a source of instant relief during an unexpected anxiety attack.

You only need to take 3 drops directly on your tongue, and your heart starts beating at a normal rate, your breath is no longer painful, and you no longer have the feeling that your breath is going to stop, and your mind starts getting clear. While you may not be totally healed immediately, the relief is incredible and it is also incredibly rapid.

The medicine is named after Richard Bach, a British physician who had observed how rural populations were able to obtain relief from the plants. Nowadays many imitations are on the market, but it's best to buy the bottles that show his name, so you can be assured of receiving the original drops.

Color Therapies

Another way of soothing if not completely getting rid of anxiety is by using colors together with energy. The therapy is known under the name of Color Therapy.

There are therapists who use this technique and apply colored stones on the patients. You may also buy a small torch and use colored papers or even colored bulbs in order to obtain the color that is necessary to help you soothe your disease. If the therapy is applied on a regular basis, your energy system will use the color to restore the flow of energy.

Emotional Freedom Techniques

Developed by Gary Craig, Emotional Freedom Techniques, also known as EFT, is a simple and powerful technique that can be applied by everyone.

EFT works with the energy blockages that cause the disease or in your case, the anxiety. It works through the meridians that are the energy highways in our body. These carry the energy across the body and these meridians are linked to our spine, or better to the channels in the back and front of our body. The energy flows through these channels and you can visualize it as transparent, white or colored. This is just to say that the main channels are located on the back and the front of the human body.

For the EFT-exercises we do not use the main channels but the points found on the hands, on the head, on the chest and under the arms. That is where the channels pass. And the blockages are located in the channels where the energy no longer flows as it should.

In order to help you with EFT, you use the fingers of one hand that will tap the karate point of the other hand, located on the side of your hand. While doing this, you say: "although I suffer terrible anxiety attacks, I love and accept myself completely and profoundly." You repeat this exercise three times. Then you tap the top of your head repeating the first part of the sentence. You do that also for three times, then you tap the area above your eyebrows, then three times at the side of your eyes, then three times under your eyes, three times under your nose, three times under your lower lip, three times under the collar bone and three times under your arms.

When you start with the first tapping, you give your emotions a value that goes from 1 to 10. Now, by tapping, you will lower this value until you feel that the anxiety is no longer so strong and does no longer hurt so much. You can repeat this exercise as often as you like. Sometimes you will feel that the anxiety grows but if you do the exercise on a regular basis, the feeling of anxiety and its invalidating side effects will diminish and you will get to overcome it completely.

The more you do the exercise, the better the results. You may change the first part of the sentence according to what you feel. The sentence or your expression may become stronger. If you do not like to say that you love and accept yourself, you may just say that you accept yourself just as you are. There are many people who, at the beginning, don't feel like saying that they love themselves. If you do not feel like saying it, you just use the second example, i.e. to accept yourself just as you are.

You can do this exercise with whatever you would like to change, but do not say that you no longer want to have the emotion of anxiety. Your subconscious mind does not distinguish between "no longer want" and "want". The negation of a sentence is not taken into consideration, in other words, if you use a negation, you will get more of what you would rather not like to get. So, be careful.

EFT has been used successfully now for more than thirty years all over the globe and, although it is so simple, the results are very good. The method is powerful.

In order to learn it properly, you may download the manual written by Gary Craig. It is free and it shows you every single step.

The Relationship Between Anxiety and Food

"He that takes medicine and neglects diet wastes the skill of the physician"—Chinese Proverb

S cientists have long ago made the connection between food and our moods. Indeed, what we eat can affect how we feel that day—and vice versa.

Most people don't recognize the relationship between food and their mental state. But as mind and body can't be separated, neither can we separate our diet from our moods. Both are strongly connected.

Too many people in our society today run to their doctor for help from pharmaceuticals to address their anxieties, only to end up with side effects, unnecessary expenses, and no sustainable relief. Little did they know that lasting freedom from anxiety and devastating mood swings could be as simple as changing their diet!

The other temptation in this fast-paced, stress filled society is to grab for all the wrong foods and beverages. Ok—so maybe you already know that what you're putting in your mouth is hurting your well being and increasing

> *Small changes can make a big difference if you're willing to give them a try.*

the bad feelings leading to anxiety and depression or worse. Maybe you fall into the bucket of people who think that eating a healthy diet requires a lot of work and expense. Maybe you think you have to give up tasty treats in exchange for more energy. Or maybe you're envisioning yourself searching endlessly for rare spices and supplements at remote health food stores. But these are all-too-common misconceptions.

Healthy foods can be found at every supermarket, and knowing just a few tips about what to eat and how to prepare nutritious meals and snacks may turn you from a junk-food junkie into a health-food junkie! Small changes can make a big difference if you're willing to give them a try.

In the following sections, you'll find information about food that will calm your nerves amidst the chaos of your most stressful days as well as overall tips for a healthier diet. The more natural energy you provide your body through a healthy diet, the better you'll be able to cope with life's demands and enjoy the pleasures available each and every day!

How Food Affects Mood

Knowing what to eat is just as important as when you eat them. But first, it is important to note how our behavior towards food plays a role in our eating habits.

Do you eat when you are anxious, regardless whether you're hungry or not? How much do you eat when you do? And what do you eat?

Most of us have a habit of eating junk food when we are sad, or drinking one cup of coffee after another when we hit a slump in our day. We have food binges, thinking it will make us feel better, when in fact it makes us feel worse.

Often, it turns into a cycle: we feel bad, so we eat junk food. We feel worse, so we eat more junk food. When it doesn't work, we start getting feelings of anxiety or despair: why am I sad? Why can't I feel better? Is something wrong with me? Why won't anything work?

Millions of people turn to food to rid themselves of their anxiety and depression. They use food as a crutch, and what's worse is that they use the wrong kind of food to do it.

You feel trapped in your situation, helpless and hopeless in the fact that nothing makes you feel better. Your fear for your condition escalates to anxiety, which slowly sinks into depression. And since it's what you usually do, you reach for the nearest stash of junk food and binge to feel better, starting the cycle all over again.

Seems familiar? Good, because now you know that you are not alone.

Millions of people turn to food to rid themselves of their anxiety and depression. They use food as a crutch, and what's worse is that they use the wrong kind of food to do it.

Breaking the Cycle

Before you learn what to eat, you must first figure out *why* you're eating.

Most of us eat when we're sad, because that's what we've been conditioned to do.

Try this experiment. Open your television and surf through your favorite sitcom. Pay attention to where the characters usually go when they have a bad day. Nine out of ten, they head to the kitchen, pouring their hearts out over a tub of ice cream.

Why do we do this? The answer is pretty simple: *because it feels good.*

Eating when we're hungry gives us instant satisfaction, something which we hope to replicate when we're sad. Like children, we gravitate towards sugary treats because it tastes good. The accompanying sugar rush also reinforces that slight high that we get immediately after eating our stash.

What we do not expect is how that sugar high can cause our energies to slump at the end of the day, leaving us tired, depressed, and anxious because our session with food did not work.

So the next time you feel low, stop and evaluate before you head off to the kitchen. There are other ways when to make yourself feel better other than breaking a bar of chocolate, such as exercise or meditation, either of which can leave you just as satisfied as having a full meal.

A Daily Regimen for Success

The most important thing is to eat a good breakfast. Remember what the word "breakfast" means: you're breaking the "fast" that your body has been enduring since your last meal the night before.

> *The most important thing is to eat a good breakfast.*

Breakfast gives you the fuel you need to start your body's engine and rev up your metabolism, which provides the foundation for your day.

Breakfast: Try eating a good cereal without any added sugar, and add yogurt or some milk for additional protein. A cereal containing barley doesn't irritate your nervous system and can actually enhance your mood. A freshly pressed juice gives you vitamins and natural sugar. Include some nuts and if you like, eat one egg. Eggs are protein-rich and contribute to the production of neurotransmitters that are responsible for making us feel alert and energetic.

Morning Snack: Eat a piece of fruit or a handful of nuts mid-morning for a natural energy boost rather than grabbing for that second or third cup of coffee. Almonds are great stress relievers as they are packed with vitamin B2, vitamin E, magnesium and zinc. Zinc has been shown to fight some of the negative effects of stress while vitamin E is an antioxidant that destroys the free radicals that can lead to stress and heart disease. They can help you get in a good mood or help you to keep it!

Lunch: At lunch every option is open as long as it does not contain foods that are too fatty or too salty. Avoid eating chips. French fries can be eaten on occasion. They are less fatty and less salty than chips, which are nothing but empty calories. But get in the habit of adding a salad to all your main meals since it will fill you up and provide fiber and nutrients at the same time. You can find ready-to-consume salads everywhere. They are washed and just need some dressing. An easy and healthy dressing can be a yogurt. It adds some proteins and a little fat to your greens.

Afternoon Snack: In the afternoon it's tempting to grab for a bar of chocolate or a cookie or a caffeinated drink when you feel that 3:00 PM "slump." Try an experiment for a week by grabbing for a healthy source of energy instead

You will feel better and think more clearly with some slight adjustments in your daily eating habits. You're worth it!

one that won't add empty calories or give you a burst of energy followed by a crash. The afternoon is a good time to try a natural fruit juice (canned juices contain too much refined sugar), nuts, or a piece of cheese with some sliced vegetables. You will feel better and think more clearly with some slight adjustments in your daily eating habits. You're worth it!

Evening: In the evening, a light meal will do. There is a saying that goes: "Eat breakfast like a king, lunch like a prince and dinner like a pauper." Eating the bulk of your calories early in the day starts you off with more energy and gives you a chance to burn off calories to sustain your metabolism. Heavy foods eaten in the evening can be hard on your digestive system and might interfere with your sleep. Grilling meat or veggies for dinner is an easy way to prepare fantastic meals without a lot of effort. Grilled dishes do not need high amounts of fat. They can be seasoned with herbs to boost their flavor. You can also add flavor and vitamins if you use lemon juice.

Lemon is one of the best natural flavor enhancers. It helps up-grade the flavor of meats, fish and veggies. It also adds flavor to your drinking water and to strawberries. Add it to other berries or fruit salads rather than adding extra sugar. Even your green salads can be made tastier with some drops of lemon juice. Lemon juice also helps your digestion and at the same time it enhances your immune system. Lemons are available everywhere.

So you see, you can eat healthier without spending more time or money than you do now. And remember that we eat with our eyes as well as our mouths! If something looks colorful and is prepared in an attractive way, it will actually taste better and be more fun and healthier to eat than something you don't like to look at. With a little bit of creativity you can prepare dishes that look good and taste even better!

Comfort Foods that Cause Discomfort

In the event that you do find yourself in the general direction of the kitchen, it is important to know what foods to eat to make you feel better, and which to avoid.

One surprising discovery is that most of the things we considered comfort food can actually make us feel worse, rather than better!

Chocolate and Everything Sweet

Chocolate, cakes, ice cream and all other sugary treats in-between lead the list of things we should stay away from when we're anxious or depressed. Since they taste good, we gravitate to sugary foods first to make us feel better, and the accompanying sugar rush gives us a temporary high. Alas, it is also the same sugar rush that will have your body crash and burn a few hours later.

Most people who indulge at work usually feel listless and fatigued during the middle of the day, making it more difficult for them to focus on tasks. This, in turn leads to poor performance and low job satisfaction, leaving you frustrated with your work.

Those who indulge late in the evening, right before bed, find that they have difficulty sleeping. The sugar rush stays on long after you're ready to go to bed, robbing you of a few hours of rest.

Fortunately, you don't have to give up chocolate altogether. Taken in moderation, chocolate can actually make you feel good. A quarter of a candy bar should be enough to flood your brain with endorphins, but not enough to give you that sugar rush.

Healthy Alternative:

If you feel like satisfying your sweet tooth, why not try eating fruit?

Fruits taste just as sweet without too much sugar content, preventing that sugar rush. The water content found in fruits aids in digestion and speeds up your metabolism, leaving you feeling light and energetic.

Craving for some ice cream? Have a sorbet instead! The lack of cream takes away that heavy feeling you get from eating ice cream, letting you have a cold and sweet treat without much sugar and calories.

Coffee and Soda

Let's face it, some of us aren't even human unless we've had that first cup of coffee in the morning. Others don't even start functioning until they're on their third cup, drinking more throughout the course of the day. If not coffee, others rely on soda to keep them perked up.

The main ingredient found in coffee and other fizzy drinks is a natural stimulant called caffeine, which can cause heart palpitations. The effect for some can be so bad, that people often confuse them with panic attacks. Couple this with the accompanying sugar rush, and it might just trigger an anxiety attack.

Since most people view caffeinated beverages as harmless, those who are prone to panic or anxiety attacks never make the connection. Coffee and soda are also regularly consumed during meetings or when faced with a late-night deadline, making an already stressful situation worse.

Caffeine, like cigarettes, is also addictive, so some feel angry and irritable when they don't have their fix. Giving up caffeine should be done gradually and in stages, as not to trigger withdrawal symptoms or mood swings.

In drinking caffeinated beverages, those prone to anxiety or panic attacks should pay close attention to when they have their symptoms. Increased heart rates, sweaty palms and ringing in your ears are reactions *after* drinking soda or coffee is the result of having too much caffeine, *not* an anxiety attack.

Still, hope is not lost for coffee lovers. The anti-oxidants in coffee have been found to prevent cancer, providing you drink it in moderation.

Healthy Alternative:

Instead of drinking coffee, why not try having some herbal teas or tonics instead?

A cup of cinnamon tea can spice up your day without any caffeine. Want something more exotic? Try boiling ginger in water for ten minutes, and drinking the infusion. Another popular product is teas or tonics with ginseng, which can boost your energy without sending your heart racing.

Instead of drinking coffee, why not try having some herbal teas or tonics instead?

Alcohol

Alcohol is a natural depressant. Although it can make you feel calm and sedate in the short term, it can also be dehydrating. That's the reason why drinking too much results in a hang-over. A hang-over is your brain's reaction to losing water, so if you don't keep yourself hydrated when you drink, you get a nasty headache a few hours later.

The dehydration caused by alcohol consumption can often exacerbate anxiety for those who are prone to having anxiety or panic attacks. The accompanying depression contributes to their feeling of helplessness, resulting in more feelings of frustration.

So next time you're in a bar, keep the alcohol to a minimum, or none at all.

Healthy Alternative:

Drink lots of water! It may not seem as chic, but opting for club soda (or a Shirley Temple) and skipping on that second or third glass of margarita will make you feel better—and your head will thank you the day after.

Water not only cleanses your system, but regular hydration ups your metabolism. If you would like something with more pizzazz, there are several brands that now offer flavored water without any of the sugary guilt that go with it.

If you would like a drink to calm you down, drink milk. Tryptophan, which is found in milk, can help produce serotonin and the amino acid melatonin, which helps you sleep.

Fast Food and Processed Food

Make it a point to eat more natural things as possible. You never know what chemicals are found in processed food that might be contributing to your bad mood. Most processed foods are high on salt and preservatives, leaving you feeling heavy and bloated.

> ## *Make it a point to eat more natural things.*

Likewise, greasy fast foods make you feel heavier and sluggish, which in turn makes you sleepy during your work day. This can lead to frustration over your inability to focus on your job, which can then lead to more stress.

Healthy Alternative:

Pack your lunch! Not only will you know what exactly goes into your food, but you'll be amazed at the amount of money you'll be able to save.

You can also control the amount of spices that go into your food, making it taste better. The better it tastes, the more satisfied you'll feel, leaving you to feel fuller. Thus, having you eat less, and not more.

Wheat and Dairy

Wheat and dairy are considered by some as highly allergenic foods, or food that normally cause allergic reactions in people.

Food like cheese or whole wheat bread and pasta sometimes provoke minor allergic reactions, which are largely associated to mood fluctuations.

The best way to test this is to observe your reactions to food containing wheat or dairy. Try going on a wheat and dairy free diet for two – three weeks, and then gradually re-introduce them. See if there is a marked difference in the way you feel, or if it triggers any food allergies that you were otherwise unaware of.

Healthy alternatives:

Non-wheat bread or pasta is now available in most health food stores, as well as soy cheese and soy milk, as a replacement for its dairy counterparts.

Healthy Snacks:
Foods to Improve Your Mood

"Let thy food be thy medicine."—Hippocrates

Everybody likes to snack. And nowadays, most people are aware that the best snacks are small and nutritious and serve to give you energy in between regular meals. They should never serve as the meal itself and should not be filled with empty calories, industrial sugar or simple carbohydrates. But not everybody knows how to choose snacks that are nutritious, easy to prepare and easy to eat at the same time.

One mistake people make when changing their diets is that they focus on subtracting, not adding to the list of things they already eat.

One mistake people make when changing their diets is that they focus on subtracting, not adding to the list of things they already eat.

Ideally, young people should have access to healthy snacks from an early age so they'll get used to eating properly, and will naturally enjoy foods like fruits, veggies, yogurt, cream cheese, rye bread and other healthy foods.

49

It's also important to remember that we all eat with our "eyes" as well as our mouths! When a snack looks colorful and interesting, it is more appealing to both children and adults.

A little bit of effort can go a long way in helping your family enjoy their healthy snacks. Below are some ideas for healthy snacks that are easy to make, appealing to the eye, delicious and "easy" on the pocketbook.

Try adding these to your diet:

Fruit Kabobs

Cut fruit into small pieces and then put them on a stick like a kabob. Alternate the fruit with rye bread until the stick is complete.

This snack gives you vitamins and some carbs. It does not contain fats and no sugar except for the fruit sugar.

You can use any type of fresh fruit as long as it doesn't contain any syrup that can leak out and make the bread soggy.

Turkey-Vegetable Kabobs

Another healthy snack that contains proteins are pieces of cooked turkey that you also put on a stick. You can alternate them with small slices of cucumber or another veggie that you like.

This snack does not contain sugar at all and very little fat, but does contain some fibers and proteins.

Veggie/Fruit Dips

A healthy snack that appeals to both children, and the kid in you too, is a fruit or vegetable "dip." Cut up your

favorite vegetable or fruit and serve them with a healthy dip such as plain yogurt.

This snack gives you some vitamins, a little fat and protein. Resist using fat-free products as they usually contain some additives that are not healthy at all.

Rye Crackers with Cream Cheese Dip

Another option for a healthy snack could be rye crackers with a dip of cream cheese. Select a brand of cream cheese that contains low salt or is salt-free.

Cream cheeses with low salt content are available everywhere. If you love cream cheese, you will be thrilled by the idea of eating some crackers together with this cheese. Rye crackers are a good choice as they are more nutritious than many wheat-based crackers.

Fruit-Vegetable Kabobs

These kabobs can be made with pieces of fruit that you alternate with pieces of veggies, all of them put on a stick like a kabob.

This is a very low calorie snack but is colorful and appealing to the eye.

Experiment with different combinations of healthy foods for your snacks and have fun with them. Everything you eat can support your body, improve your mood and give you the vitality you need to enjoy your life!

Nuts

Nuts are rich in Omega-3 essential fatty acids, a type of fat that allows mood-lifting neurotransmitters to function properly.

We have to remember that our brain is made mostly of fat, so avoiding fat altogether can be dangerous. In fact, diets low in Omega-3 essential fatty acids can lead to depression, anxiety, and a host of other mental problems.

Nuts are rich in Omega-3 essential fatty acids, a type of fat that allows mood-lifting neurotransmitters to function properly.

So next time you're feeling blue, open a packet of walnuts, or have a peanut butter and jam sandwich to help boost your mood.

Other foods with Omega-3 essential fatty acids are:

Seeds and fish. Tuna, mackerel, and salmon are rich in Omega-3 essential fatty acids.

For a quick fix, you can also drink cod liver oil. Not only is it rich in Omega-3 essential fatty acids, but it also contains vitamins A and D. Cod liver oil is also available in pill form, so check out your local health food store for your options.

Oatmeal

Oatmeal is considered a good carbohydrate, which releases Tryptophan. It is a good carbohydrate because unlike other carbs, it is slow releasing and thus absorbs Tryptophan better, preventing that sugar crash associated with a sudden influx of carbs.

Since oatmeal is a slow releasing carbohydrate, it also releases energy evenly throughout the day, allowing you feel better longer. The lack of the sugar crash also takes away the anxiety and mood fluctuations associated with it, allowing you to focus on work with renewed energy and vigor.

Oatmeal, like fruit, is also a great alternative to having sugary treats. An oatmeal cookie not only gives you energy, but the high fiber content cleans out your digestive tract.

Lentils and Spinach

There's a reason why Popeye feels better when he has spinach!

Spinach and lentils are a natural resource of Vitamin B, which produces foliate, another acid that helps produce serotonin.

Foliate helps ease clinical depression, and lowers our anxiety levels, keeping us feeling sunny and healthy for the rest of the day.

A salad filled with lentils and spinach is a good end to a meal, because they are also water vegetables. Water vegetables help stimulate digestion, so eating a salad after a meal instead of before helps metabolize your meals better.

There's a reason why Popeye feels better when he has spinach!

You can also try making lentil soup, which is light enough that there's not much to digest, and also adds to your water intake.

A Diet that Makes You Feel Better

Most people shudder at the thought of having a diet, and worry about how they will accomplish eating less.

This type of diet focuses on what you eat, and when, rather than how much. Our behavior towards food varies with our mood, and the effects are even more with anxious people.

Some use food as a crutch, eating more to make them feel better, finding that sense of satisfaction that you can only get when you're full. Binge eating only results in gaining weight and eating the wrong foods, resulting in mood swings and weight fluctuations.

Others do not eat at all, thinking that limiting their meals will also limit their anxiety, giving them a sense of control. This robs your brain of vital nutrients that are necessary to help regulate your mood.

By knowing what you eat and how it affects you, you will begin to notice a change in your mood not possible in your old lifestyle. Not only will you feel more in control, but you will feel more optimistic about things.

Staying away from foods that can trigger your anxiety is just one step from breaking that cycle of hopelessness and depression.

Natural "High"
or Fast-Food Junkie?

"If we're not willing to settle for junk living, we certainly shouldn't settle for junk food."—Sally Edwards

How often do you go to a fast food restaurant? Do you also know how many calories you take in with a normal fast food meal? It is probably more than you think. It might even be the total amount of calories you should take in all day long. All those sandwiches, breads, sauces, meats and bacon: it adds up! And the piece of lettuce and slice of tomato hardly provide the serving of vegetables you should be having with every meal. They are practically with no calories.

"But I eat chicken at fast food restaurants," you say. "Isn't chicken supposed to be good for you?" Chicken by itself may be low in calories, but in many fast food restaurants you get fried chicken, covered with bread and deep fried in oil, which is extremely high in calories. And what do you eat with fried chicken? French fries!

French fries are one of the worst fast food "offenders." These are usually prepared with low quality oils, and often with "exhausted" oils: oils that have been used many times to deep fry whatever came their way. If you prepare your meals at home, you can eat French fries once in a while because you can be sure you're using fresh, quality oil. But you should avoid eating them at restaurants on a regular basis.

Another often-encountered junk food is hamburgers. Again, they are deep-fried and the quality of the meat is often very bad. The problem with junk food is not the essential components. In fact, if taken separately, the ingredients of fast food may even be "natural" food. It is the way they are treated, processed and cooked which turns them into junk food.

If you cooked your potatoes in a steamer or had them transformed into hash browns, they certainly would not be junk food but would be rich in fiber and nutrients. The same can be said of hamburgers. You could cook the individual parts of the hamburger mixture, separating the meats and cooking them as short fried meat to eat together with pasta. Add a fresh tomato instead of ketchup, and you'd end up with a satisfying, healthy meal.

And it can go on and on.

But what do you do when you're away from home and you need a fast meal?

Nowadays you can eat a mixed salad, a bowl of soup and even have some bread. You don't really need to put butter on it as the bread already has a good taste, and may even be made of non-wheat grains. You can even eat a fruit salad that adds fiber without adding refined white sugar. In most cases, the sugar is just that of the fruits themselves. You can also choose to eat the fried chicken with a mixed salad. This combination helps you to better digest the fat of the fried food as the salad contains bitter leaves.

If you drink a glass of milk, you could choose a lower calorie skimmed milk. Instead of juice, just have plain water.

That is what your body needs. And, you may be surprised that it is also the favorite drink of your brain. In fact, your brain needs water in order to work well.

You see, a fast food restaurant meal does not need to be high calorie food. It is your choice whether you want the high calorie food with its implications for your body or whether you prefer the health-friendly low calorie food. Or try a combination of both to see if you can make some small changes over time to turn you from a junk food junkie to a health food fan!

B Vitamins and Anxiety

"You are what you eat—so don't be fast, cheap, easy or fake."—Author unknown

Don't forget that anxiety may be a normal reaction in stressful situations. It only becomes a problem if you feel it all day long. Then it is no longer a normal reaction but has become a habit. Your anxiety may result from the fear of an anxiety attack, which becomes a repeating cycle that perpetuates itself. When anxiety becomes a habitual reaction, it has to come to an end, or you might harm yourself and your overall health.

In any case, who wants anxiety for a companion? It is not a very good friend! You need to develop new "friends" through a healthy way of living, which includes giving your body the vitamins it needs to protect you against the negative effects of your anxiety.

Be aware that the most important vitamins your body needs when it is anxious are those of the B-group. They all have a strong impact on your psyche, your mental state, and your nervous system.

First of all, be aware that the most important vitamins your body needs when it is anxious are those of the B-group. They all have a strong impact on your psyche, your mental state, and your nervous system.

Every single vitamin of this group plays a particular part in maintaining your nervous system in good health.

Vitamin B1: also called thiamine. This vitamin improves your mood. It is important in keeping the heart and the nervous system running normally. A lack of this vitamin can cause irritability. Sometimes it also influences your energy level.

Vitamin B2: also called riboflavin. It is required by the body to produce anti-stress hormones. It also helps to release energy stored in food. Furthermore, it is needed for the metabolism of proteins.

Vitamin B3: also called niacin. Its deficiency causes mental instability. Anxiety and stress can cause skin related problems. This vitamin provides a protection against skin problems and inflammation.

Vitamin B5: helps the body produce anti-stress hormones. As anxiety is strongly related to stress, the lack of these vitamins could cause your anxiety to show up more often.

Vitamin B6: also known as pyridoxine. It has a role in keeping your nervous system functioning properly. If you are ingesting insufficient amounts of B6, you might experience anxiety or even depression, insomnia and/or irritability.

Vitamin B12: plays a big role in providing the necessary brain chemicals that make you feel good. This vitamin is also essential for the production of red blood cells.

There are other types of vitamin B that are still being studied in relation to their beneficial effects on your health, but to date, every single vitamin B is involved in the proper functioning of the nervous system, which in turn, directly affects your mood. If you prefer to feel calm and peaceful instead of anxious and irritable, don't forget your B vitamins!

Most of these vitamins are available in their natural form in the diets of most cultures that include meat or other animal proteins. It is recommended that vegans, therefore, supplement their diet with B12.

There are many sources for the whole group of B vitamins:

B1: wheat germ, peanuts, pork and brown rice

B2: milk, yogurt, avocados, beef liver

B3: chicken, potatoes, sunflower seeds

B5: eggs, avocados, nuts, green vegetables

B6: bananas, fish, chicken, seeds in general and cabbage

B12: all animal proteins

You can certainly cover your needs for vitamin B if you take into consideration the various foods available in your area. By eating the right food you can protect yourself against anxiety. If you already suffer from anxiety, you can lessen its frequency or intensity by eating the appropriate food and ensuring you're ingesting proper levels of B vitamins.

Anxiety and Spicy Food: Subtract the spices to add to your peace

"Eat food. Not too much. Mostly plants."
—Michael Pollan, An Eater's Manifesto

Spicing foods is an age-old tradition in many cultures. The spices that became "traditional" for a given culture were influenced by climate and the native spices that were locally available. It was also an issue of hygiene, as a number of "hot" spices are strong disinfectants, and in fact, are most often eaten in countries with hot climates.

As populations became more mobile, expatriating and moving to countries far from their homeland, they took their culture with them, including their traditional foods and spices. This was probably a good idea since they were used to their own dietary habits physically, mentally and emotionally. This made the food easier to prepare and easier for their systems to digest.

Over time, they started to mix with the indigenous population and develop new habits that brought about all sorts of changes. They got used to eating other foods and seeing other cereal and fruit crops, and no longer did they stay within the boundaries of their own dietary traditions. They slowly developed new eating habits over the course of years and decades, which gave their bodies a chance to adjust naturally to the introduction of new foods and spices.

If you suffer from anxiety, be mindful of the impact of the abrupt change your body might experience when you eat spicy foods.

Fast forward to present day, and not only can you eat dishes of various cultures as you travel all over the globe, you can choose from many ethnic restaurants within a few city blocks! There are whole shelves devoted to foods that are traditional for different cultures within a single supermarket. There have never been so many dietary choices at our fingertips.

This is good news and bad news. It's exciting to have the opportunity to easily sample the cuisine of a different culture each night of the week if you desire, but it can also wreak havoc on your system, which hasn't had the opportunity to adjust naturally to dietary changes.

If you suffer from anxiety, be mindful of the impact of the abrupt change your body might experience when you eat spicy foods. Spicy foods are often referred to as "hot" because they dilate your blood vessels, causing blood to flow towards your throat and head. This can cause you to feel hot and flushed, start to sweat and also increase your heart rate. As such, these physical signs are not dangerous, but if you're prone to anxiety, they can exacerbate your symptoms. This can be a scary feeling and will certainly ruin your meal!

If you already suffer from anxiety or tend to have a strong reaction to unusual food ask yourself whether spicy food really belongs to your culture. If it doesn't, do yourself a favor and don't eat it! Stick to your own cuisine. Spicy food should be enjoyed once in a while, but not on a regular basis if it isn't part of your culture. Make a note of any food that increases your anxiety and try to avoid it in order to live a more tranquil life. If you DO have an attack of anxiety, at least you'll know that it wasn't caused by your dinner!

Black Sesame Seeds: Add a Spice to Decrease Your Anxiety and Rebuild Your Body and Spirit

"But I love spicy foods," you say. Ok— I have the perfect option for you: black sesame seeds.

Black sesame seeds are a very old spice, maybe the oldest one in the world. Their earliest recorded use as a spice is traced back thousands of years. According to an Assyrian legend, the gods drank sesame-based wine before they created the earth! And they are still a main food source and spice in every part of Asia and in some parts of Europe and Africa.

Sesame seeds as such, come in various colors, but not all of them offer the same benefits as black sesame seeds, which are dark in color, small and flat. Although they are considered a culinary treat, they are often used for their medicinal properties since they have a very high content of minerals primarily calcium and iron.

According to Chinese medicine, black sesame seeds have sweet and neutral properties. What does this mean? How can they help you? They help to tone up "yin," the female energy of the human body. And they help build the spirit, which is of utmost importance, not only for anxiety sufferers but for all of us. The spirit is our life force that helps us to go ahead in our life.

Black sesame seeds can be of the utmost importance in our lives, as they are associated with the liver and the kidneys. Our physical life force is based on the kidneys, so if our kidneys do not work well, our physical life force gets weak. The liver is the other "cleansing" organ of our body, and is critical for toxin elimination. If either the kidneys or liver is impaired in any way, toxins can build up in the body, raising anxiety levels and leading to other more serious disorders.

The intake of black sesame seeds helps our body to cleanse itself by flushing out toxins. Anxiety sufferers usually have all sorts of toxins in their body. If they regularly eat black sesame seeds, the elimination of those toxins is no longer a problem. They also promote regular bowel movements, so they can help people who suffer from constipation. However they should be used with caution or not at all in individuals with loose bowel movements.

Black sesame seeds also contain high amounts of protein, phosphorus and magnesium and are often recommended in cases of serious illness as they help rebuild the body and the spirit.

Black Sesame Seeds: Where to Obtain and How to Prepare

Black sesame seeds are available at herbal shops, health shops, Asian markets, and some food stores that sell exotic spices. They are also available in other forms like powder, pills or capsules. As their taste is slightly sweet and nutty, I suggest eating them in their original form. Soak 2-3 teaspoons of seeds in plenty of water, then remove the remains on the surface (empty hulls, etc.) Throw the water away and cook the seeds for five minutes in a cup of water. Then let them settle and eat them, if possible, early in the morning before breakfast. You may prepare a larger quantity (i.e. for one week) and keep it in the refrigerator. If you add these seeds to your daily food, you will soon be aware of their value and of the overall improvement in your mood and your health and well-being.

Best Fruits for an Energy Boost

"Keep as near as ever you can to the first sources of supply—fruits and vegetables."—B.W. Richardson

With all the stress we take in every day, and the anxieties that come from daily living that make us feel tired and drained, we need something to boost our energy that is as natural as possible. The perfect solution: fruit!

Many cultures are fortunate to have many fruits to choose from, and most of them can give us a natural boost to our energy, along with high amounts of vitamin C. But that is not all they give us. Most of them contain other vitamins and are also rich in water soluble fibers. Water soluble fibers are incredibly valuable: they help us digest our food and give us more nutrients, while at the same time they work to clean our intestines, which raises our energy levels.

Fruits are really an excellent choice. It's no wonder that the Britons say, "an apple a day keeps the doctor away!" They are probably right, since apples supply a healthy dose of vitamin C: a good fighter against free radicals and a booster to keep your immune system healthy. There is a great variety of apples. Not all of them contain the same amount of vitamin C, but all of them are valuable. They also give you natural fruit sugar, pectin and good fibers, which are important for your digestion. And apples are readily available, from supermarkets to the airport, to railway stations and even from apple sellers on the streets.

Then there are oranges and kiwifruit. Both provide you with vitamin C. Oranges and all kinds of red fruit also supply carotenes that are not only antioxidants but are also an initial form of vitamin A which is beneficial for your eyes. Red colored fruits include grapes, strawberries, and various other kinds of berries. Please keep in mind, however, that berries are difficult to store and should be eaten as soon as you buy them. An alternative is to buy them deep-frozen. They keep their properties during the process of deep-freezing and if you warm them up slowly you can enjoy them as if they were fresh.

Dried fruits are easy to store and can be combined with unsalted nuts such as peanuts, walnuts or almonds to create an easy, colorful and healthy snack. They offer a concentrated source of vitamins, minerals and antioxidants. Commonly found dried fruits include cranberries, apples, pineapple, bananas, cherries, mangoes, and raisins. You can even find dried peaches and cantaloupe in some

> *A very valuable fruit is the date. It contains various vitamins, minerals, trace elements and sugar.*

supermarkets and natural food stores. Dried fruit is a natural energy booster and can also be a healthful alternative to refined sugar for those with a sweet tooth. Be mindful as you bite into the chewy goodness of dried fruit. Take your time, letting the flavors burst onto your tongue. You'll see just how satisfying dried fruit can be!

A very valuable fruit is the date. It contains various vitamins, minerals, trace elements and sugar. You could live on a few dates a day if you had to. You wouldn't suffer from any deficiencies and wouldn't even feel hungry.

Bananas are very rich in magnesium and potassium. They can further contribute to your energy level because they also contain carbohydrates and sugar.

When you live in an exotic country you will have many fruits that are not available in the USA or only at an expensive price. It's best to eat local fruits. If this is not possible, eat the fruits that have not traveled long distances to arrive onto your table.

Foods that Promote a Healthy Bowel

"Plant a radish, get a radish, never any doubt.
That's why I love vegetables, you know what
they're about!"—Tom Jones and Harvey Schmidt

Though many of us don't like to talk about it, one of the biggest contributors to anxiety is the inability to have a healthy, normal bowel movement. The more trouble we have, the more anxious we get, which in turn impacts the health of our bowel; we either have loose bowel movements or none at all, leading to chronic constipation. Both conditions can be helped with the proper intake of fiber.

Do you know how important these fiber-rich foods are? Are you aware of how poor most foods are? Many are poor in fibers. The problem is more wide spread in western countries where a lot of processed food is consumed. Most people do not eat enough fresh fruit and vegetables. Eating the recommended amount of fresh fruits and vegetables on a daily basis would give us the necessary fibers and would dramatically improve the health of our bowels and our overall mood.

Fibers that help your bowel movements are also found in lentils, in beans of all kinds and in nuts. Certain seeds are especially helpful if you suffer from constipation, including flax seeds and sesame seeds. Some dried fruit can also help you solve the problem.

But let us face the situation in order.

Breakfast: Start your day with a glass of lukewarm water. Sip it slowly. The best way to get the optimum lukewarm water is by boiling half of the water and filling up the glass with cold water. The two waters together create a lukewarm water and are built with different molecules, thus giving the water a cleansing effect. By not drinking anything cold to start with, your body is not shocked. After your glass of so-called "yin-yang" water (warm and cold mixed together,) you can eat your normal breakfast. Ideally, rather than drinking the traditional glass of juice, include a whole fresh fruit, which provides more of the natural fiber needed for a healthy bowel.

Morning Snack: Instead of eating a cookie in the course of the morning, have an apple or another seasonal fruit.

Lunch: Include a salad and other vegetables whenever possible. Season it lightly with a little salt, a little pepper, some vinegar and some oil. Use olive oil if possible. If you are used to having a dessert after your normal lunch, choose natural, unsalted nuts. Peanuts, walnuts and cashew nuts are all good choices.

Afternoon Snack: If you are used to having a snack in the afternoon, you may have a cookie, but it's best if it is made of grains of oat that provide more fibers.

Dinner: Build more fiber into your dinner by including salad and adding as many different boiled vegetables as possible. Vegetables that are properly boiled until they are soft will aid your digestion. Try to avoid broiled vegetables. They are difficult to digest and their fibers might even disturb you after your meal in contrast to the boiled vegetables that can help you.

Your bowel movements are of the utmost importance. They help eliminate what the body cannot use. They help cleanse your system and keep you healthy. Therefore, pay attention to your food and keep in mind that fiber rich food is essential to your mood and to your overall well-being.

Best Foods for Fresh Breath

"Don't eat anything your great-grandmother wouldn't recognize as food."—Michael Pollan

When we are feeling stressed or anxious, sometimes our own self-care suffers. But the last thing you want to do is add to your stress by wondering if you have breath that may be offensive to others and feels stale to yourself.

Bad breath can have various causes, including disorders of the stomach and intestines; however, the majority of causes are related to how you treat your teeth and mouth, and are the easiest to fix!

Your first step to fresh breath is to pay attention to your teeth, your gums and your mouth.

Brushing your teeth regularly is a rule. Using small brushes and floss to clean the spaces in between the teeth is an absolute must since even the best and healthiest food can leave traces in between the teeth and create bad breath.

Some Yogurt a Day Keeps Bad Breath Away!

What really causes bad breath are the bacteria that develop either in your mouth or in your digestive tract, but this can be treated with simple means with something as easy to eat as yogurt. Yogurt is a fermented dairy product made by adding bacterial cultures to milk. They produce lactic acid, giving yogurt its tart flavor and thick texture.

> *Yogurt has so many health benefits that in many grocery stores, it has practically taken over the dairy aisle.*

Yogurt has so many health benefits that in many grocery stores, it has practically taken over the dairy aisle. Not only do you get a dose of animal protein, because yogurt comes from milk, but the "active bacteria cultures" used in the fermenting process contain probiotics. Probiotics are "friendly bacteria" that are naturally present in the digestive tract and are needed for optimum health.

Studies have shown that consuming just 3.2 ounces of yogurt (90 grams) twice a day not only lowers the levels of hydrogen sulfide and other sulfide compounds responsible for bad breath, but may also eliminate bacteria that coat the tongue, reduce dental plaque formation that might also cause bad breath, and reduce the risk of cavities and gingivitis. It is believed that the live bacteria in the yogurt overcome the sulfide-producing bacteria in the mouth.

The best yogurts indicate exactly how many live cultures are contained in the product. The most commonly found cultures contain lactobacillus bulgaricus, streptococcus thermophiles and bifidobacteria. Different strains of these bacteria produce different flavors and may have slightly different effects on your body. The best idea is to try several different brands to determine the one that suits you best.

Herbs for Fresh Breath

Parsley and dill are well known for their high chlorophyll content and both serve as great mouth fresheners. Since parsley is often used as a garnish on your plate when you're out to eat, you can readily take advantage of this "free breath mint" by chewing on this herb after your meal. Feel free to swallow it, it will keep your breath fresh for hours! Dill also has digestive and diuretic properties, so it serves to enhance any meal.

Other herbs that you can either eat or simply chew after a meal or throughout the day include coriander, spearmint, cardamon and tarragon. If you use fresh herbs, you can also put them into hot water and drink them like a tea. These not only combat halitosis, but are excellent digestives. So you get a double benefit!

Vitamins for Fresh Breath

Eat food that contains vitamin C. This vitamin creates an inhospitable environment where bacteria cannot survive. Vitamin C containing foods include oranges, lemons, limes, grapefruit, broccoli and other green leafy vegetables such as spinach. You don't necessarily have to ingest supplements because vitamin C is present in many other foods not even mentioned here. Pepper, for example, is a good source of vitamin C and of flavanoids that help your skin and your blood circulation.

The Best Dessert for Good Health and Good Breath!

Another way to clean your mouth after a meal is eating an apple. In fact, the juice contained in the apple is able to clean your teeth. And it cleans them thoroughly. The juicy apple, like a Granny Smith, helps you to overcome your problem. And, after all, as already noted, an apple a day keeps the doctor away!

Her Majesty—the Potato

"You don't have to cook fancy or complicated masterpieces—just good food from fresh ingredients."—Julia Child

You may smile and ask yourself, "Why is this simple produce considered a queen? A majesty?" Many people don't give the potato the respect it deserves. I am going to show you why it gets the title of a noble plant.

First of all, the potato is the number one vegetable crop in the world. It is known almost everywhere and eaten in various styles. This plant belongs to a group called nightshade plants. This group includes tomatoes, eggplants, peppers and tomatillos. They are the swollen part of the underground stem, called a tuber. The tuber is designed to provide food for the green leafy portion of the plant. If this plant is allowed to flower and the flower becomes a fruit, it resembles a tomato, but cannot be eaten.

The potato offers numerous health benefits. Unfortunately, most people eat potatoes as French fries or potato chips, both full of grease and fat. Even baked potatoes are not consumed in their natural state, but are typically filled with butter, sour cream, melted cheese or bacon, which decreases their healthy potential.

The potato offers other astonishing qualities. It contains 60 different kinds of phyto-chemicals and vitamins in the flesh and also in the skin.

If consumed with such a heavy load of fat, the potato is a potential contributor to heart disease, including strokes and heart attacks. But take away the extra fat or the deep frying and eat it plain or seasoned with herbs, and a baked potato is exceptionally healthful. It brings low calories, a high fiber content and offers important protection against cardiovascular disease and cancer. Analyses show that they are also one of the most effective plants for lowering blood pressure.

The potato is a very good source of vitamin C, a good source of vitamin B6, minerals like copper, potassium and manganese, and as already mentioned, a good source of dietary fibers. In addition to these healthful ingredients, it contains a variety of compounds that protect against free radicals.

The potato offers other astonishing qualities. It contains 60 different kinds of phyto-chemicals and vitamins in the flesh and also in the skin, whether they're grown wild or commercially. The idea that the potato is just a "starch-giver" can definitely be abolished!

Actually, potatoes have been grown for thousands of years. They originated in the Andean mountain region of South America. It is estimated that potatoes have been cultivated by the Indians living in these areas for 4,000 – 7,000 years.

Potatoes are one of the rare plants that can be grown at these high altitudes and they therefore became a staple food for these people. The compounds are so numerous and healthful that the potato should be included in everybody's diet as long as they are not consumed just as French fries.

I hope that you now understand why the potato is called a queen. It is actually a star guest in many a kitchen around the globe!

What Artichokes Can Do
For Your Health

*"A good cook is like a sorceress who dispenses
happiness"—Isa Schiaparelli*

The artichoke is a true surprise as far as our health and our mood is concerned. Many people don't realize the many components that can assist in bringing relief from many diseases. It even presents itself in a pleasant form, as it appears like a flower. It is mainly grown in the Mediterranean region and was first mentioned by the Egyptians.

Let us start with common diseases that can be cured by the bitter contained in artichokes. This bitter is not contained in what one usually eats of the artichoke. It is extracted from the dried leaves and can be taken as a tea (soaking dried leaves in water) or in the form of pills or tablets. The bitter can bring relief from disorders of the liver and gallbladder. The bitter can increase the flow of gall so that it is sufficient to deal with the fat contained in your food.

Most people are familiar with eating the flower bud of the artichoke which is also the "heart." You can also eat the flesh from the leaves. Both include a surprising amount of nutrients and helpful ingredients that make it worthy of our attention! These include the following:

Vitamin C: aids the absorption of iron and also improves the immune system and prevents you from getting colds and flu.

Pro-vitamin A: good for your eyes

Vitamin B1 and B6: aid in proper nervous system function

Vitamin B9: also called folic acid. Its task is to produce healthy new cells in the body. It is therefore of the utmost importance.

Zinc: an essential mineral that has various tasks in the body and is therefore absolutely necessary.

Iron: very important in the building of new blood cells. Women need more of it as they lose iron with their monthly recurrence.

Calcium: needed for the bones and teeth.

Magnesium: helps build protein. Artichokes contain approximately 4% protein. This protein is very valuable because it is not linked to fat. As a vegetable protein, it is pure and can be easily absorbed.

Flavonoids: antioxidants that prevent your blood vessels from being destroyed or lined with plaque. This is very important because plaque may cause a restriction of your arteries. This means that your blood cannot flow properly and nourish your brain or other parts as it should.

In addition to the conditions and benefits noted above, the artichoke is an excellent help in case of joint pains and metabolic diseases. If your hips hurt so much that you can hardly walk, the nutrients of the artichoke may be able to help reduce your aches and pains.

So eat them often. Enjoy their delicate taste and thank Mother Nature for this gift.

Small Changes Add Up to Big Improvements

"One of the very nicest things about life is the way we must regularly stop whatever it is we are doing and devote our attention to eating"—Luciano Pavarotti

I hope by now you're convinced that our diet makes a difference. What we eat affects how we feel and how we feel affects what we eat. When we're feeling stressed or anxious, we may have a tendency to overeat or under-eat or eat the wrong foods. All these choices are hard on our bodies the very bodies that are trying their best to support us!

Be kind to yourself and make self-care a priority by examining your diet and picking one or two small changes to make on a weekly or even a monthly basis. Don't try to make major changes all at once, particularly when you're suffering from anxiety or depression or both. Pick one idea from this book and make a commitment to give it a try for 7-10 days. The very act of

> *Pick one idea from this book and make a commitment to give it a try for 7-10 days.*

making even one, small, healthy choice sends a message to your body, your mind and your spirit that you are willing to make the changes you need to feel better and that you're ready to take back control of your life.

Ask yourself the following questions. You don't have to answer them all. Just pick one that resonates with you and see what answers come to mind as you "chew" on it for a little while.

1. What aspects of my diet are working well for me and help me to feel good? What do I want to keep on doing?

2. What one aspect of my diet do I know I need to change in order to feel better? How can I make it fun and easy to make that change?

3. Which meal do I pay the most attention to? What can I do to make that meal more healthful?

4. Which meal do I tend to neglect? How can I improve that meal in order to take better care of myself?

5. What is one unhealthy snack that I currently eat that I'm willing to replace with a healthy snack? What would taste good to me?

6. Who else can support me in making the changes I need to make in my diet?

7. How am I going to celebrate once I've incorporated some healthy changes in my diet?

Don't discount the need to celebrate and reward yourself as you make the dietary changes you need to support your health and vitality. Change can be difficult when you're feeling stressed or overwhelmed, yet it's absolutely necessary. They say the definition of insanity is "doing the same thing and expecting different results." Likewise, you can't keep eating the same things and expect to feel any differently. So, plan to reward yourself in a healthy way once you've formed some new, healthy eating habits: buy some flowers, take a loved one to a movie, relax with that new book you've been wanting to read, or invite some friends over for a healthy meal that you've cooked yourself.

Don't discount the need to celebrate and reward yourself as you make the dietary changes you need to support your health and vitality.

Eating well can be easy and fun and is the FIRST thing to consider when you're feeling anxious not the LAST. Good food really can put you in a good mood. Try it you're worth it!

What About Exercising?

"I think if you exercise, your state of mind—my state of mind—is usually more at ease, ready for mental challenges. Once I get the physical stuff out of the way it always seems like I have more calmness and better self-esteem."—Stone Gossard

Have you ever seen the movie "Legally Blonde"? Interning law student Elle Woods came up with this unbelievable defense in a murder trial where the accused is a fitness instructor: *"Exercise gives your body endorphins. Endorphins make people happy. Happy people don't kill their husbands!"*

While the logic is exaggerated for comedic effect, there is more than a grain of truth in Elle's argument. Regular physical exercise has natural comforting properties. Exercise has been known not just to help with depression, but with anxiety as well.

Exercise as a Natural Tension Reliever

Exercise gives your body endorphins—the natural anti-depressant. Aside from endorphins, exercise also releases serotonin, norepinephrine, and dopamine. These are neurotransmitters that influence the mood and help fight off diseases.

The results have been documented. A research conducted by Dr. Andreas Stroehle, an Assistant Professor of Psychiatry from Charite-University Medicine Berlin, found that physical exercise has acute anti-panic effects. In fact, when the effects of a quiet rest versus a 30 minute aerobic treadmill exercise were compared, it was found that prior exercise results in significantly lower panic attacks.

> *Exercise gives your body endorphins— the natural anti-depressant.*

The effect of exercise on a person is not just via endorphins. Aside from physical improvement, it gives mental benefit as well.

Exercise as Bodily Meditation

The mental hygiene principles that we discussed earlier also apply to physical exercise.

Physical exercise forces your mind to focus: it is about getting the best performance that you possibly can despite tiredness or exhaustion. It's also about dedicated persistence.

> *Focus and persistence are important skills to learn when you are struggling with anxiety.*

Focus and persistence are important skills to learn when you are struggling with anxiety. Often, anxious people have difficulty following through a regular exercise regimen because of their fears and apprehension, similar to how difficult they may find experiencing anxiety. By learning focus and persistence to get to a goal in physical rather than mental threat, they develop the sense of achievement they can call on when they get an anxiety attack.

Finding Yourself Through Meditation

Taking a few minutes of each day for yourself is enough to clear your mind, but if you find it hard to concentrate, try meditating to music.

Some find that listening to the sounds of waves crashing or gentle rain falling soothes them. Others need more direction, so a track with *What is important in meditation, is to be consistent.* a person guiding them to relax is ideal. There are CDs available for purchase at most music stores, or available to download off the Internet.

What is important in meditation, is to be consistent. You must try to find the time to relax everyday. To break the monotony, try doing different exercises: listening to music one day, doing breathing exercises for another. It can even be as simple as taking a long, hot bath at the end of the day.

Also, some people have some difficulty meditating while they are just sitting or standing still. When you exercise, you can make your body movements as a focal point of meditation. In this sense, exercise is a way of transcendence. While you exercise, your mind and body are temporarily free from the usual demands placed upon them.

That physical exercise can be a form of meditation is something Oriental remedies have taken advantage of. Most

Chinese and Japanese exercises, for example, are meditative in nature.

One of these methods is QiGong. QiGong is a traditional Chinese exercise that combines physical movements with regular breathing with the goal of focusing on particular energy centers in the body.

Traditional QiGong may be difficult for the typical Westerner to appreciate. For this reason, Westerner-friendly versions of these methods have been formulated. One of these versions is called the SpringForest QiGong. This method was developed by a Chinese Master residing in USA who understood that the Ancient QiGong methods which have been in use for thousands of years in China, are no good for people in the industrialized countries because they are too complicated and the Chinese mentality is not understood so easily. This Master is Chunyi Lin.

Chunyi Lin says that this method is based on love, forgiveness and kindness. These three concepts of life help live a good life. According to Chunyi Lin, and I invite you to prove it to yourself, that a smile relaxes the whole body. It really is very true. If you practice it daily, whenever you can, you will immediately get the benefit of a relaxed body. If your muscles are relaxed, anxiety has no chance.

If you are interested in learning SpringForest QiGong, there are courses, manuals, cassettes/ cds available in specialist centres in the state of Minnesota and through LearningStrategies.com and through the SpringForestQiGong online-shop.

Exercise as Natural Detoxification

Few people know that exercise is a good detoxification method. Even in the mere fact that you get to sweat, your body is already releasing toxic chemicals in your body.

Susceptibility to anxiety can possibly be the effect of the many toxins that are in your system.

Exercise also stimulates our lymphatic system. This means that the more we move around, the better able our body can deliver oxygenated blood to the different organs in our body. When all our vital

Few people know that exercise is a good detoxification method. Even in the mere fact that you get to sweat, your body is already releasing toxic chemicals in your body.

organs are functioning optimally, we are less likely to feel the tension in the different parts of our body.

Simple Exercises That You Can Do at Home or At Work

A lot of people equate exercise as going to the gym. Although there's nothing wrong with signing up for the gym, the commitment for some can be overwhelming—and an excuse not to exercise.

There are others ways to get your exercise *without* leaving your home, or even eat hours of your time.

It is best that you have a regular time allotted to do exercise. But if you can't, there are many ways that you can incorporate physical exertion in your daily routine.

Walk

If your office is near your workplace, opt to walk rather than drive a car or commute. Walking, alongside with jogging, is considered as the most popular and the most detoxifying exercise. A daily 15-minute walk can result in significant health improvement. Remember that it is better to walk outside in fresh air so opt rather for an outdoor exercise than an indoor one as much as you can.

Try walking the dog for half an hour, or taking the stairs instead of the elevator on your way up to work. If you're based at home, pick up a few cans of fruit and start doing shrugs. Search on the Internet for running clubs in your area.

For higher impact and greater socialization, try picking up a new sport, or teaching one at your local Boys and Girls Club.

Simple Stretches

Walking is an aerobic exercise—it is to help your heart and your lungs. But exercise is not just for aerobic purposes, they are also there to relax your muscles and increase your flexibility. Whenever you can, take the time to stretch your body. This is especially true if you work an office job that necessitates you sit down the entire day.

Some of the simple exercises that you can do at work or at home include: stretching your arms high in the air as far as you can reach and then gradually setting it down to you back; bending down and reaching for your toes with your knees straight; squatting in your seat and standing up repeatedly.

Standing Up

Yes, standing up! Researches reveal that you actually burn more calories standing up than sitting down. It helps therefore that you find ways to stand up as much as you can. If you work in an office, answer the phone standing up, pace if you can do so. Making this a habit can already help you a lot.

Do You Really Want Your Health Back?

*"What do you first do when you first learn to swim? You
make mistakes do you not? And what happens?
You make other mistakes, and when you have made
all the mistakes you possibly can without drowning—
and some of them many times over—what do you
find? That you can swim? Well, life is just the same
as learning to swim! Do not be afraid of making
mistakes, for there is no other way of learning
how to live!—Alfred Adler*

A real choice is not a one time deal; it is a choice that
you have to make over and over again.

Living with anxiety can be difficult, but it doesn't have
to be a curse, nor does it have to be forever. By making
simple changes to your lifestyle, you are well on your way
to regaining your health.

Still, the path to recovery is not easy. The exercises
and diet tips outlined in this book are not miracle cures,
but guidelines to help you on your journey back to health.
Practicing them requires a lot of work and discipline, and
there will be days when you will forget or make mistakes.
That is not important. What is important is your commitment

> *The exercises and diet tips outlined in this book are not miracle cures, but guidelines to help you on your journey back to health.*

to saying goodbye to anxiety, and getting your life back on track.

So ask yourself: *do you really want your health back?*

If so, how much do you want it? The answer will determine how much you are willing to adapt these changes to your life, and how long you are willing to stick with it.

Instead of making a giant leap, take smaller steps to ease yourself into the new routine.

The following are a few suggestions on how to help you make that transition:

Getting Your Health Back... in 21 Days

They say habits can be formed in 21 days. This means that in three weeks, you can either develop new habits, or get rid of old ones.

Taking that first step towards change is always the most difficult one, so here are a few guidelines that can help you get on your way:

1. *Make a list of what you want to change.* Ask yourself why you are undertaking this journey, and what for? By listing your goals, you not only make them more visible, but more achievable.

2. *Write down a battle plan.* Having a schedule can help you stay on course, and make the next few days a lot less overwhelming. Plan your meals for the next three weeks, and detail what exercises you will be doing and when. Reserve certain times of

the day for meditation, and inform your family ahead of time to limit unnecessary interruptions.

3. *Keep a journal.* It may seem like you're doing an awful lot of writing, but it is important to note what triggers your feelings of anxiety and when. Knowing what causes these episodes not only helps in eliminating them, but it will make you feel more in control of your life, something which you haven't felt in a long time.

4. *Have an accountability partner.* The first few days of making the transition will be difficult, so you may need to talk to someone who is aware of what you're going through. It can be someone from your family, a friend, or a counselor. These people will also serve as your "living reminders", helping you focus on changing your lifestyle and staying on track.

Even if you get through the three weeks smoothly, there may be some times when you might slip back to your old habits. That's okay; just ease back into your new routine. Stumbling is part of the process.

Always remember that these first three weeks are just a building block to your way to recovery, one that is naturally healthy and anxiety free!

> *There may be some times when you might slip back to your old habits. That's okay; just ease back into your new routine. Stumbling is part of the process.*

About the Author

Elisabetta Reist works with clients of all ages to release anxiety and experience the peace and joy that come from being freed from emotional traumas. Her personal journey to peace led her to achieve certification as an instructor of EFT, EmoTrance, Remap, Agegate Therapy and SpringForest QiGong.

Elisabetta is dedicated to sharing the tools and techniques she discovered on her own journey to break the cycle of anxiety that had kept her trapped for years. This book is the result of her research into the relationship between nutrition and anxiety and the results that are possible with a healthy, life sustaining diet.

Elisabetta provides customized coaching in English, Italian, German and French to help clients release limiting beliefs and achieve their dreams. She can be reached through Skype @ elisabetta.reist1 or via email: ereist@ reistlingue.com.

Visit her websites: *http://www.stopanxietyquick.com* and *http://www.kissanxietygoodbye.com* for more information on how you can let GO of anxiety in just 21 days and live the life of joy and peace you deserve.

Are you ready to start to feel better now? Go to either site and download your FREE report on The Quickest and Easiest Ways to Reduce Your Anxiety and immediately access your FREE meditation recording under the "Meditation" tab. You'll be glad you did!

References

Bradshaw, John (1988). *"Healing the Shame that Binds You"* USA: Health Communications, Inc.

Coué, Emile (1922) *"Selfmastery though Conscious Autosuggestion"* Library for Higher Learning and Personal Development Institute.

Craig Gary, www.emofree.com

Greary, Amanda. (2001). *"The Food and Mood Handbook: Find Relief at Last from Depression, Anxiety, PMS, Cravings and Mood Swings"*. Thorsons.

Master Chunyi Lin, SpringForestQiGong, Eden Prairie MN/ USA, www.springforestqigong.com; www.bornahealer.com

McGraw, Philip C. (2001). *"Self-Matters: Creating Your Life from the Inside Out"* USA: Simon & Schuster

Pratt, Charlotte W. 85 Cornely, Kathleen (2004). *"Essential Biochemistry"* USA: John Wiley and Sons.

Scheele, Paul, www.LearningStrategies.com

Schultz, Johannes, Luthe Wolfgang: *"Autogenic Therapy: Volume 1, and "Autogenic Therapy"* Volume II: Medical Applications

Somer, Elizabeth (2004). *"The Food and Mood Cookbook: Recipes for Eating Well and Feeling Your Best"* USA: Henry Holt and Company

Taylor, C. Barr 85 Arnow, Bruce (1998). *"The Nature and Treatment of Anxiety Disorders"* USA: The Free Press.

For Your Notes

For Your Notes

For Your Notes